MILADY'S STANDARD: NAIL TECHNOLOGY EXAM REVIEW

Compiled by Deborah Beatty

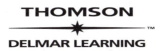

THOMSON

™

DELMAR LEARNING

Australia   Canada   Mexico   Singapore   Spain   United Kingdom   United States

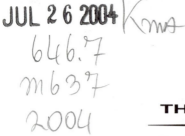

THOMSON
DELMAR LEARNING

Milady's Standard: Nail Technology Exam Review, Fourth Edition
Compiled by Deborah Beatty

Library of Congress Cataloging-in-Publication Data
ISBN 1-56253-909-4
TT958.3 .M55 2002
646.7'27—dc21   2002075308

NOTICE TO THE READER

Publisher does not warrant or guarantee any of the products described herein or perform any independent analysis in connection with any of the product information contained herein. Publisher does not assume, and expressly disclaims, any obligation to obtain and include information other than that provided to it by the manufacturer.

The reader is expressly warned to consider and adopt all safety precautions that might be indicated by the activities herein and to avoid all potential hazards. By following the instructions contained herein, the reader willingly assumes all risks in connection with such instructions.

The Publisher makes no representation or warranties of any kind, including but not limited to, the warranties of fitness for particular purpose or merchantability, nor are any such representations implied with respect to the material set forth herein, and the publisher takes no responsibility with respect to such material. The publisher shall not be liable for any special, consequential, or exemplary damages resulting, in whole or part, from the readers' use of, or reliance upon, this material.

Contents

This book of exam reviews contains questions similar to those that may be found on state licensing exams for nail technology. It employs the multiple-choice type question, which has been widely adopted and approved by the majority of state licensing boards.

Groups of questions have been arranged under major subject areas. To get the maximum advantage when using this book, it is advisable that the review of subject matter take place shortly after its classroom presentation.

This review book reflects advances in professional nail technology. It attempts to keep pace with, and insure a basic understanding of, sanitation, anatomy, physiology, and salon business applicable to the nail technician, client consultation guidelines, chemical safety in the nail salon, and basic manicuring and pedicuring procedures as well as some of the more advanced and creative aspects of the profession.

The book serves as an excellent guide for the student as well as for the experienced nail technician. It provides a reliable standard against which professionals can measure their knowledge, understanding, and abilities.

Furthermore, these reviews will help students and professionals alike to gain a more thorough understanding of the full scope of their work as they review practical performance skills and related theory. They will increase their ability to evaluate new products and procedures and to be better qualified professionals for dealing with the needs of their clients.

chapter 1

YOUR PROFESSIONAL IMAGE

Directions: Carefully read each statement. Insert on the blank line after each statement the letter representing the word or phrase that correctly completes the statement.

1. The way you behave toward others when working in a salon is called:
   a) good will
   b) professional ethics
   c) salon conduct
   d) behavior _____

2. If you keep to your appointment schedule, clients will think you are:
   a) fast
   b) competent
   c) unusual
   d) lazy _____

3. The time to set up your station and sanitize your instruments is when clients are:
   a) getting coffee
   b) not yet present
   c) waiting
   d) in the bathroom _____

4. Your daily schedule should include clients' names so that you can:
   a) greet them by name
   b) plan your tips
   c) get larger commissions
   d) arrange for parking _____

5. When your appointments are running slightly late, your arriving clients should:
   a) reschedule
   b) expect shortcuts
   c) be informed
   d) go home _____

6. Your attitude toward clients should always be:
   a) courteous
   b) crisp and businesslike
   c) arrogant
   d) gossipy _____

7. To make them feel welcome, new clients should be:
   a) greeted by name
   b) given a salon tour
   c) escorted to a station
   d) all the above _____

8. Mrs. Smith is always hard to please; today, she's especially difficult. In dealing with her, you should:
   a) act professionally
   b) ask her to leave
   c) yell
   d) charge her more _____

9. When you are around nail chemicals, it is dangerous to:
   a) wash your hands
   b) chew gum
   c) talk loudly
   d) smoke _____

10. When you communicate with your employer, no matter what the subject, you should always be:
    a) grateful for the job
    b) honest
    c) assertive
    d) asking for a raise _____

11. Your employer notices a technique you use that was developed and taught to you by a coworker. In this situation, you should tell your employer:
   a) it's your technique
   b) a coworker developed the technique
   c) you learned it at school
   d) nothing—keep quiet _____

12. To get along with coworkers, you should:
   a) respect their opinions
   b) use deodorant
   c) buy their lunch
   d) point out their mistakes _____

13. If you have a problem or question about your job, you should discuss it with:
   a) a coworker
   b) a prospective employer
   c) your employer
   d) a client _____

14. Personal problems should always be:
   a) shared with coworkers
   b) shared with clients
   c) left at home
   d) told to the boss _____

15. Learning about other services offered at the salon, such as hair and skin care, and then telling your clients about them, is called salon:
   a) performance
   b) show-off
   c) networking
   d) promotion _____

16. Your sense of right and wrong when you interact with clients, employer, and coworkers is called:
   a) honesty
   b) professional ethics
   c) guilt
   d) moodiness _____

17. Your best source of advertising to get new clients is:
   a) radio
   b) current satisfied clients
   c) newspapers
   d) coupon mailers _____

18. High ethical standards towards clients (giving them only the services they need and/or want) will earn you:
   a) larger commissions
   b) the boss's approval
   c) a good reputation
   d) big tips _____

19. You have a client who is always willing to try anything you suggest. At her next appointment, you should give her:
   a) only the needed services
   b) every expensive service
   c) a discount
   d) a free polish _____

20. Your state has new regulations for sanitation and safety. You feel many of these are unnecessary as well as inconvenient, so you:
   a) comply, it's law
   b) ignore them
   c) follow some
   d) quit manicuring _____

21. Some clients love to share with you stories about your coworkers, your employer, or others in your community. When these clients start to gossip, you should:
   a) join in
   b) close your eyes
   c) leave the area
   d) remain businesslike _____

22. For tips on keeping hands beautiful between manicures, clients will ask the advice of:
   a) the nail technician
   b) a coworker
   c) a neighbor
   d) a doctor _____

23. You must learn the differences between salon and drugstore products in order to convince clients:
    a) to purchase higher-priced products
    b) to get the best deal on products
    c) that professional products are best for nail health and beauty
    d) that drugstore products lack quality _____

24. When you and your coworkers practice professional ethics, your salon will become:
    a) well-known
    b) successful
    c) more profitable
    d) less efficient _____

25. Professional ethics includes keeping your:
    a) records accurately
    b) tips secret
    c) promises
    d) breaks frequent _____

26. If a client complains to you about another technician, you should:
    a) get defensive
    b) suggest the client and technician talk
    c) tell your opinion
    d) call the boss immediately _____

27. You should be a model of good grooming because you are:
    a) self-disciplined
    b) a member of the beauty industry
    c) a pleasant person
    d) a model _____

28. For the best professional appearance, you should be clean and fresh by bathing or showering and using a deodorant:
    a) daily
    b) once a week
    c) morning and night
    d) twice a month _____

29. The clothes you wear for work should be:
    a) very dressy
    b) spot-resistant
    c) trendy
    d) professional _____

30. Female nail technicians should wear makeup to work:
    a) for special occasions
    b) once a month
    c) every day
    d) heavily applied _____

chapter 2

BACTERIA AND OTHER INFECTIOUS AGENTS

1. One-celled microorganisms that are so small they can only be seen through a microscope are called:
   a) bugs
   b) parasites
   c) fungi
   d) bacteria   ____

2. Because bacteria are so small, to cover the head of a pin you would need this many of them:
   a) 2
   b) 1,500
   c) 5 million
   d) 10 million   ____

3. Bacteria multiply rapidly. A single bacterial cell can produce 16 million more in only:
   a) two weeks
   b) three minutes
   c) half a day
   d) five days   ____

4. FDA stands for:
   a) Federal Drug Agency
   b) Food and Drug Administration
   c) Food, Drug, and Alcohol
   d) Federal Detective Association   ____

5. CDC Stands for:
   a) Control Demonstration Center
   b) Center for Dependent Children
   c) Centers for Disease Control
   d) Center for Development Career   ____

6. OSHA stands for:
   a) Occupational Self-Health Association
   b) Occupational Standards for Hepatitis and Aids
   c) Organization of Sanitation and Health Administration
   d) Occupational Safety and Health Administration   ____

7. The best defense against infectious diseases is:
   a) knowledge
   b) relying on government agencies
   c) not being concerned
   d) not understanding the causes   ____

8. Some nonpathogenic bacteria help in:
   a) improving the fertility of soil
   b) producing food and oxygen
   c) breaking down food in digestion
   d) a, b, and c   ____

9. Nonpathogenic bacteria make up the majority of all bacteria, which is about:
   a) 60%
   b) 70%
   c) 50%
   d) 100%   ____

10. Pathogenic bacteria are also called:
    a) microorganisms
    b) cells
    c) germs
    d) toxins   ____

11. Disease-causing bacteria are:
    a) aseptic   c) beneficial
    b) non-pathogenic   d) pathogen   _____

12. Round, pus-producing bacteria are called:
    a) cocci   c) influenza
    b) circular   d) mites   _____

13. Baccilli are the most common bacteria, producing diseases
    such as tetanus, tuberculosis, and:
    a) backache   c) diphtheria
    b) measles   d) cold sores   _____

14. The common name for the disease caused by treponema pallida is:
    a) toothache   c) strep throat
    b) syphilis   d) palsy   _____

15. A mature bacterial cell divides into two identical cells; this division is
    called:
    a) mitosis   c) diplococci
    b) cilia   d) spirilla   _____

16. Two types of bacteria which propel themselves are
    bacilli and:
    a) diplococci   c) cocci
    b) staphylococci   d) spirilla   _____

17. Disease-causing agents smaller than bacteria are:
    a) viruses   c) miniatures
    b) microbes   d) germs   _____

18. Viruses enter healthy cells and:
    a) die   c) reproduce
    b) remain the same size   d) leave without damaging
                                 the cell   _____

19. The disease AIDS is caused by a:
    a) spirilla   c) fungus
    b) virus   d) spore   _____

20. The transfer of the HIV virus is through:
    a) sneezing   c) touching
    b) the common cold   d) bodily fluids   _____

21. Nail fungus usually appears as a discoloration on the nail that
    spreads toward the:
    a) cuticle   c) nail bed
    b) tip   d) center   _____

22. Early stage bacterial infection can be identified as a spot which is
    colored:
    a) black   c) yellow-green
    b) blue   d) purple   _____

23. Clients with fungus or bacterial infection should be treated by a:
    a) manicurist   c) cosmetologist
    b) optometrist   d) physician   _____

24. The removal of artificial nails from a client with nail fungus or
    bacterial infection should be accomplished wearing:
    a) a gown   c) a mask
    b) gloves   d) goggles   _____

25. The ability of the body to resist a disease is called:
    a) rickettsia   c) organisms
    b) infection   d) immunity   _____

26. After the body fights off a disease, the bloodstream contains:
    a) antibodies   c) pathogens
    b) germs   d) viruses   _____

27. Vaccines are given to artificially produce:
    a) disease   c) immunity
    b) fever   d) allergies   _____

28. Bacteria and germs multiply rapidly on:
    a) nail files   c) towels
    b) cuticle nippers   d) a, b, and c   _____

29. Tiny, multicelled organisms that live off living matter without giving benefits in return are:
    a) parasites   c) viruses
    b) toxins   d) cilia   _____

30. The nail technician with a contagious common illness should:
    a) stay home   c) drink juice
    b) work quickly   d) take naps   _____

31. It is easy to wound a client by filing too deeply or when:
    a) removing polish   c) nipping cuticles
    b) massaging toes   d) applying tips   _____

32. Clients who fear being infected need to be:
    a) referred to a physician   c) distracted
    b) reassured about safety precautions   d) given health magazines to read   _____

33. Clients are interested in knowing:
    a) where disinfectants are stored   c) how they are at risk
    b) who cleans the salon   d) how you prevent the spread of disease in the salon   _____

34. To create a feeling of security in clients, give them specific examples of:
    a) disinfectants used   c) diseases that can be prevented
    b) disinfection procedures   d) treatments for nail diseases   _____

35. Factors that contribute to the spread of infectious diseases are:
    a) poor hygiene   c) poor diet
    b) broken skin   d) a, b, and c   _____

36. Nail technicians fall into the category of:
    a) social workers   c) independent workers
    b) service workers   d) medical workers   _____

37. In regard to spreading diseases, a person who looks and appears healthy:
    a) does not present a risk   c) may present a risk
    b) always presents a risk   d) is always healthy   _____

38. An important prevention in the transfer of disease is:
    a) rinsing hands with cold water   c) washing hands with liquid soap
    b) using bar soap   d) not washing hands at all   _____

SANITATION AND DISINFECTION

Chapter 3

1. Sanitation rules are legislated and enforced for:
   a) health and safety reasons   c) statistics
   b) lower insurance rates   d) keeping busy   ____

2. To destroy all bacteria and make something germ-free is to:
   a) sanitize   c) deodorize
   b) clean   d) sterilize   ____

3. To significantly reduce the number of pathogens on a surface is to:
   a) sterilize   c) wash
   b) sanitize   d) bleach   ____

4. Antiseptics help prevent:
   a) spread of viruses   c) skin infections
   b) soft nail tips   d) cracked nails   ____

5. Disinfection does not kill:
   a) germs   c) the HIV virus
   b) bacterial spores   d) fungus   ____

6. A disinfectant should not come into contact with:
   a) implements   c) cabinets
   b) table tops   d) skin   ____

7. The Material Safety Data Sheet provides all the following except:
   a) directions for proper use   c) pricing information
   b) a list of active ingredients   d) safety precautions   ____

8. Implements will contaminate disinfecting solution if they are:
   a) dirty   c) warm
   b) wet   d) dry   ____

9. A glass receptacle which holds disinfectant and a submerged implement is called a/an:
   a) glass   c) disinfection container
   b) agent   d) antiseptic   ____

10. Cloudy solution in a disinfection container indicates:
    a) contamination   c) strong solution
    b) weak solution   d) ammonia   ____

11. According to the EPA, implements should be fully immersed in disinfecting solutions:
    a) for three minutes   c) for at least 10 minutes
    b) until they are clean   d) for twenty minutes   ____

12. The most commonly used disinfectant in salons is:
    a) formaldehyde   c) quats
    b) bleach   d) phenolics   ____

13. The most expensive disinfectants are:
    a) alcohol and bleach
    b) phenolics
    c) antibacterial soaps
    d) quats ____

14. Alcohol loses effectiveness as a disinfectant when diluted below:
    a) 62%
    b) 70%
    c) 75%
    d) 85% ____

15. After disinfecting counter tops, you should:
    a) let them air dry
    b) leave the room for three minutes
    c) wipe them with a clean towel
    d) sponge away excess disinfectant ____

16. When using a spray bottle for disinfectants, you should wear:
    a) a hairnet
    b) a gown
    c) an apron
    d) a vapor mask ____

17. Before touching sanitized implements, the nail technician's hands should be cleaned with:
    a) ammonia
    b) bleach
    c) liquid soap
    d) formalin ____

18. Disposable items are to be discarded after use:
    a) on two clients
    b) on one client
    c) on five clients
    d) at the end of the day ____

19. Following disinfection, dry implements should be stored
    a) in a jar
    b) in your pocket
    c) according to your state regulations
    d) in a paper towel ____

20. Bead "sterilizers" should not be used because:
    a) they are ineffective
    b) they are a waste of money
    c) they pose health risks
    d) a, b, and c ____

21. Formaldehyde is a/an:
    a) safe disinfectant
    b) commonly used fumigant
    c) recommended disinfectant in all states
    d) allergic sensitizer ____

22. To prevent the release of fumes from products used in artificial nail applications, upon completion:
    a) light a candle
    b) run air conditioner
    c) discard in a covered trash container
    d) spray air freshener ____

23. Tuberculocidal disinfectants are recommended for cleaning:
    a) rest rooms
    b) blood spills
    c) doorknobs
    d) counter tops ____

24. If you accidentally cut a client with a file, you should:
    a) immediately wash the file
    b) give the client the file
    c) put disinfectant on the cut
    d) send the client home ____

25. When mixing or using salon products, you should:
    a) wear gloves and safety glasses
    b) measure everything carefully
    c) read and follow instructions exactly
    d) a, b, and c ____

26. Pouring disinfectant on your hands can:
    a) decrease the chance of infection
    b) protect your skin from pathogens
    c) cause skin disease/disorders
    d) promote good health ____

27. Store professional products:
    a) in a cool, dark, dry location
    b) on low shelves within easy reach
    c) in a well-lit closet
    d) under the sink ____

28. Universal Sanitation includes all of the following except:
    a) wearing gloves
    b) using disinfectants
    c) taking short cuts
    d) sanitizing the salon ____

29. All of the following affect nail health except:
    a) pregnancy
    b) weight
    c) diet
    d) prescription drug use ____

30. You can custom-tailor a manicure to solve an individual's problems if you are:
    a) knowledgeable about nail health
    b) fashion-conscious
    c) consulting with a doctor
    d) using an airbrush ____

chapter 4

SAFETY IN THE SALON

1. Lightheadedness, runny nose, and tingling toes are symptoms of chemical:
   a) burn
   b) inhalation
   c) overexposure
   d) exposure
   ____

2. A Material Safety Data Sheet will tell you about a product's potential:
   a) price increase
   b) hazards
   c) reformulation
   d) discontinuation
   ____

3. An MSDS must include information about all of these areas except:
   a) first aid procedures
   b) physical hazards
   c) protection measures
   d) application methods
   ____

4. Carcinogens are substances that can cause:
   a) skin irritation
   b) cancer
   c) flash fires
   d) spoilage
   ____

5. An MSDS can be obtained from your salon's:
   a) distributor
   b) main office
   c) cleaning person
   d) fire department
   ____

6. OSHA mandates that each business fulfill specific requirements regarding:
   a) training
   b) inventory control
   c) written procedures for handling hazardous material
   d) a, b, and c
   ____

7. OSHA mandates that a complete inventory of products be kept:
   a) for quick reference
   b) for clients to read
   c) to take up space
   d) to occupy the receptionist's time
   ____

8. According to the labeling mandates by OSHA, all containers must:
   a) be clearly labeled
   b) be intact and accurate
   c) contain appropriate warnings
   d) a, b, and c
   ____

9. Nail product chemicals enter your body in all these ways except:
   a) inhalation
   b) ingestion
   c) injection
   d) skin contact
   ____

10. Proper ventilation requires that fumes and vapors be vented to:
    a) the reception area
    b) the bathroom
    c) outside the building
    d) the haircolor area
    ____

11. An exhaust system should completely ventilate and replace the air volume treatment area:
a) 2-4 times per hour   c) 10-12 times per week
b) 4-6 times per hour   d) 6-8 times per hour   _____

12. To be effective, the charcoal filter in a vented manicuring table must be changed every:
a) week   c) 48 hours
b) 20 hours   d) month   _____

13. The area the size of a beach ball that is directly in front of your mouth is:
a) your allergy zone   c) your health zone
b) your breathing zone   d) your ventilation zone   _____

14. You can eliminate vapors by all methods except:
a) tightly sealing product containers   c) running fans
b) avoiding the use of pressurized sprays   d) emptying waste containers   _____

15. The best solution to salon vapor and dust control is:
a) fans   c) local exhaust
b) a vented manicure table   d) air cleaners   _____

16. The distance between a roof exhaust pipe and an intake vent should be at least:
a) eight feet   c) fifteen feet
b) ten feet   d) twenty-one feet   _____

17. An accidental splash of disinfectant solution or primer can seriously injure the:
a) nail   c) implements
b) manicure table   d) eyes   _____

18. To protect the lungs when filing nails, you and your client should wear:
a) dust masks   c) oxygen tanks
b) bandanas   d) clean towels   _____

19. Dust masks quickly lose their effectiveness and should be replaced:
a) every few days   c) monthly
b) daily   d) yearly   _____

20. When the possibility for chemical splashing exists, you and your client should wear:
a) masks   c) rubber aprons
b) gloves   d) eye protection   _____

21. Because of the possibility of eye injury, contact lenses should not be worn when:
a) skiing   c) working in the salon
b) swimming   d) showering   _____

22. Many nail products are highly flammable; thus, smoking near them could cause a:
a) ventilation overload   c) skin allergy
b) fire   d) chronic cough   _____

23. To avoid ingesting chemicals at your station, you and your clients should not:
    a) smoke
    b) breathe
    c) touch
    d) eat or drink

24. Food and chemicals in the salon should be stored in:
    a) the refrigerator
    b) paper bags
    c) separate areas
    d) the office

25. To help prevent chemical ingestion, never eat anything in the salon without first:
    a) washing your hands
    b) asking permission
    c) having an antacid
    d) taking a sample

26. To prevent chemical accidents, never use a product if its container is not:
    a) sealed
    b) sanitized
    c) full
    d) labeled

27. Storage for chemicals should be in cool areas and away from:
    a) any appliance/furnace with a pilot light
    b) hair colors
    c) perm solutions
    d) garbage cans

28. Nail products can be ruined by:
    a) overmixing
    b) excessive heat
    c) shaking too hard
    d) cool temperatures

29. Many nail products are even more flammable than:
    a) oils
    b) charcoal
    c) water
    d) gasoline

30. To help keep your area well-ventilated, empty your trash containers:
    a) daily
    b) weekly
    c) several times per day
    d) monthly

31. Capping products will reduce vapors and make them:
    a) look neater
    b) last longer
    c) harder to open
    d) easier to steal

32. To cover the small dishes you use for acrylic powder and liquid, use:
    a) jar lids
    b) marbles
    c) plastic wrap
    d) aluminum foil

33. Cumulative trauma disorders can be caused by all these factors except:
    a) chemical overexposure
    b) repetitive motion
    c) awkward twisting
    d) working in one position

34. To turn safety into a promotion for nail art, add your hand-painted designs to the frames of:
    a) safety goggles
    b) nail dryers
    c) dust masks
    d) chairs

NAIL PRODUCT CHEMISTRY SIMPLIFIED

Chapter 5

1. Sulfur cross-links create strong:
   a) natural nails
   b) toxins
   c) odors
   d) vitamins _____

2. Energy has no:
   a) velocity
   b) heat
   c) substance
   d) power _____

3. A water molecule can be broken down into:
   a) helium and oxygen
   b) hydrogen and oxygen
   c) hydrogen and ozone
   d) helium and ozone _____

4. When water becomes ice, there is a:
   a) chemical change
   b) physical improvement
   c) chemical reaction
   d) physical change _____

5. A catalyst can make a chemical reaction:
   a) cleaner
   b) faster
   c) hotter
   d) slower _____

6. A substance that dissolves something is called a/an:
   a) solute
   b) enhancement
   c) catalyst
   d) solvent _____

7. When performing a basic manicure, the acetone polish remover is considered a solvent and the nail polish is considered:
   a) a solid
   b) saturated
   c) a solute
   d) a compound _____

8. When removing artificial nail enhancements, warming the solvent to 105° :
   a) speeds up the removal time
   b) slows down the removal time
   c) does not affect the removal time
   d) none of the listed _____

9. A chemical that causes two surfaces to stick together is a/an:
   a) contaminant
   b) adhesive
   c) saturated solvent
   d) surfactant _____

10. Substances that improve adhesion are:
    a) primers
    b) solutes
    c) enhancements
    d) corrosives _____

11. Washing hands and scrubbing the nail plate removes:
    a) the bacteria which causes most fingernail infections
    b) surface oils
    c) contaminants
    d) a, b, and c _____

12. Adhesion is best when the nail plate is:
    a) roughed up
    b) thin
    c) cold
    d) clean and dry
    _____

13. Overfiling the nail plate can lead to:
    a) lifting
    b) curling
    c) painful friction burn
    d) a, b, and c
    _____

14. Gigantic chains of molecules are called:
    a) corrosives
    b) monomers
    c) polymers
    d) histamines
    _____

15. When an initiator touches a monomer it:
    a) destroys it
    b) energizes it
    c) tranquilizes it
    d) disables it
    _____

16. A billion monomers can join in less than:
    a) a second
    b) five minutes
    c) thirty minutes
    d) one hour
    _____

17. A monomer that joins different polymer chains is called a:
    a) bridge
    b) rung
    c) cross-linker
    d) tie
    _____

18. Light-cured enhancements generally use:
    a) infrared light
    b) ultraviolet light
    c) visible light
    d) incandescent light
    _____

19. All of the following are evaporation coatings except:
    a) nail polishes
    b) gels
    c) top coats
    d) base coats
    _____

20. The most common skin disease for nail technicians is:
    a) acne
    b) eczema
    c) psoriasis
    d) contact dermatitis
    _____

21. Sensitive clients generally show allergic symptoms after repeated exposure for:
    a) one to two months
    b) four to six months
    c) eight to nine months
    d) ten to twelve months
    _____

22. You must always leave a margin between the skin and the product of:
    a) 1/16"
    b) 1/8"
    c) 3/16"
    d) 3/8"
    _____

23. U.V. bulbs remain blue for years but loose their effectiveness after:
    a) 1 year
    b) 1 month
    c) 4-6 months
    d) 3 months
    _____

24. Allergic reactions are caused by all the following except:
    a) overexposure
    b) improper product consistency
    c) any contact with monomers
    d) custom blending your own mixture
    _____

25. The percentage of nail technicians affected by skin disorders on their hands is more than:
    a) 40%
    b) 30%
    c) 50%
    d) 65%
    _____

26. When the skin is damaged by irritants, the immune system releases:
    a) histamines
    b) antibodies
    c) antitoxins
    d) hormones ____

27. A common salon irritant is:
    a) skin cream
    b) cuticle oil
    c) tap water
    d) rubbing alcohol ____

28. Prolonged or repeated contact with solvents will leave the skin:
    a) burned
    b) oily
    c) shiny
    d) dry and damaged ____

29. Product dusts and residues can accumulate on:
    a) brush handles
    b) containers
    c) table tops
    d) a, b, and c ____

30. In order to sell a product you should do all of the following except:
    a) insist that the client needs it
    b) use the product in the service
    c) place the item in the client's hand
    d) ask if you can add it to the ticket ____

31. The best time to attempt to sell the product is:
    a) during the initial consultation
    b) while you use the product
    c) at the end of the manicure
    d) when you schedule another appointment ____

ANATOMY AND PHYSIOLOGY

Chapter 6

1. The study of the structure of the body and what it is made of is called:
   a) physiology
   b) anatomy
   c) medicine
   d) physical _____

2. The study of the microscopic, individual structures of the body, such as hair, nails, sweat glands, and oil glands, is called:
   a) psychology
   b) anatomy
   c) histology
   d) microbes _____

3. An understanding of body structure will make you more proficient when doing:
   a) hand and arm massage
   b) basic manicures
   c) pedicures
   d) acrylics _____

4. The basic unit of all living things is:
   a) tissue
   b) protein
   c) the nucleus
   d) the cell _____

5. The protoplasm of the cell consists of all the following except the:
   a) nucleus
   b) cilia
   c) cytoplasm
   d) centrosome _____

6. The cell is surrounded by the:
   a) nucleus
   b) protoplasm
   c) centrosome
   d) cell membrane _____

7. Cells reproduce themselves through a process called:
   a) anabolism
   b) centrosome
   c) mitosis
   d) nucleus _____

8. The chemical process whereby the body cells are nourished is called:
   a) metabolism
   b) anabolism
   c) mitosis
   d) centrosome _____

9. The maintenance of normal, internal stability in the body is called:
   a) mitosis
   b) anabolism
   c) homeostasis
   d) catabolism _____

10. The protective covering on body surfaces such as skin and mucous membranes is called:
    a) muscular tissue
    b) epithelial tissue
    c) nerve tissue
    d) connective tissue _____

11. Cartilage and ligaments are examples of:
    a) liquid tissue
    b) muscular tissue
    c) fat tissue
    d) connective tissue _____

12. Messages are carried to and from the brain by:
    a) brain tissue
    c) liquid tissue
    b) nerve tissue
    d) epithelial tissue ____

13. Structures designed to accomplish a specific bodily function are called:
    a) cells
    c) organs
    b) building blocks
    d) nuclei ____

14. The number of systems in the body is:
    a) 10
    c) 15
    b) 5
    d) 25 ____

15. All of the following are bodily systems except the:
    a) integumentary system
    c) synovial system
    b) circulatory system
    d) excretory system ____

16. The physical foundation of the body is the:
    a) cell
    c) heart
    b) skeleton
    d) muscles ____

17. Bones are connected by movable and immovable:
    a) bands
    c) nerves
    b) tissues
    d) joints ____

18. The skeleton is composed of:
    a) 206 bones
    c) 50 bones
    b) 260 bones
    d) 157 bones ____

19. The skeletal system has several primary functions, including all the following except:
    a) regulating body temperature
    c) protecting internal organs
    b) acting as levers for movement
    d) storing minerals ____

20. Bone is a hard connective tissue consisting of bone cells called:
    a) periosteum
    c) phosphorus
    b) synovial
    d) osteocytes ____

21. Bones are covered by a specialized connective tissue known as:
    a) periosteum
    c) osteocytes
    b) synovial
    d) phosphorus ____

22. The bands of fibrous tissue which support the bones at the joints are called:
    a) cartilage
    c) ligaments
    b) ulna
    d) periosteum ____

23. The ankle and wrist are:
    a) pivot joints
    c) hinge joints
    b) gliding joints
    d) ball-and-socket joints ____

24. The large bone on the small-finger side of the forearm is the:
    a) clavicle
    c) radius
    b) ulna
    d) humerus ____

25. The long, slender bones of the palm and hand are the:
    a) carpus
    c) metacarpals
    b) phalanges
    d) fibula ____

26. The foot is made up of:
    a) 26 bones
    c) 28 bones
    b) 30 bones
    d) 35 bones ____

27. In the foot there are 14 bones called phalanges which compose the
    a) patella
    b) tarsal
    c) ankle
    d) toes _____

28. The muscles in the human body number more than:
    a) 100
    b) 500
    c) 800
    d) 1,000 _____

29. Muscles of the face, arm, and leg are:
    a) myology
    b) cardiac
    c) non-striated
    d) striated _____

30. Smooth muscles function automatically and are classified as:
    a) striated
    b) non-striated
    c) cardiac
    d) slick _____

31. Muscle tissue can be stimulated by all of the following except:
    a) massage
    b) infrared and ultraviolet rays
    c) nerve impulses
    d) fluorescent light _____

32. The muscle which turns the hand inward so the palm faces
    down is the:
    a) pronator
    b) supinator
    c) flexor
    d) extensor _____

33. The muscle which turns the hand outward so the palm faces
    upward is the:
    a) pronator
    b) supinator
    c) flexor
    d) extensor _____

34. The muscles which separate the fingers are called the:
    a) adductors
    b) abductors
    c) opponent
    d) flexor _____

35. The muscles which draw the fingers together are the:
    a) adductors
    b) abductors
    c) pronator
    d) flexor _____

36. The muscle attached at the rear of the heel which pulls the foot
    down is the:
    a) gastrocnemius
    b) soleus
    c) gluteous maximus
    d) peroneus longus _____

37. The muscle which covers the front of the shin and bends the foot
    upward and inward is the:
    a) soleus
    b) peroneus brevis
    c) tibialis anterior
    d) peroneous longus _____

38. The following are nervous system divisions except:
    a) autonomic
    b) cerebro-spinal
    c) neurology
    d) peripheral _____

39. Body movements are controlled by the:
    a) central nervous system
    b) peripheral system
    c) sympathetic system
    d) parasympathetic system _____

40. The sympathetic division of the autonomic nervous system is
    activated during times of:
    a) rest
    b) homeostasis
    c) stress
    d) deep thought _____

41. Nerves which carry impulses from the brain to the muscles are called:
a) afferent nerves   c) receptors
b) efferent nerves   d) mixed nerves   _____

42. The nerve which serves the fingers is the:
a) ulnar   c) digital
b) radial   d) sural   _____

43. The nerve which supplies impulses to the skin on the top of the foot is the:
a) sural   c) tibial
b) dorsal   d) saphenous   _____

44. The heart, arteries, veins, capillaries, lymph glands, and lymph vessels make up the body's:
a) circulatory system   c) respiratory system
b) endocrine system   d) digestive system   _____

45. The bodily fluid which aids in protecting the body from harmful bacteria and infection through its white cells is:
a) lymph   c) water
b) urine   d) blood   _____

THE NAIL AND ITS DISORDERS

Chapter 7

1. The technical term for nail is:
   a) keratin
   b) onyx
   c) osteo
   d) matrix ____

2. A medical doctor who is a skin specialist is a/an:
   a) dermatologist
   b) podiatrist
   c) intern
   d) cardiologist ____

3. Functions of the normal nail include all except the following:
   a) handling small objects
   b) grooming purposes
   c) protection
   d) producing heat ____

4. The normal growth rate per day of a fingernail is:
   a) 3 mm
   b) 3 cm
   c) 0.3 mm
   d) 0.1 mm ____

5. It takes 6 months to replace a fingernail and for a toenail to be replaced it takes:
   a) 3-4 months
   b) 18-24 months
   c) 6-8 months
   d) 12-18 months ____

6. Certain conditions such as psoriasis can cause the growth rate of a nail to:
   a) remain the same
   b) decrease
   c) increase
   d) none of the listed ____

7. Cold temperatures cause nail growth to:
   a) remain unaffected
   b) decrease
   c) increase
   d) increase to three times the normal rate ____

8. Nail growth rate peaks between the ages of:
   a) 12-14
   b) 10-14
   c) 21-23
   d) 45-50 ____

9. The normal nail unit is composed of:
   a) 3 basic parts
   b) 6 basic parts
   c) 8 basic parts
   d) 2 basic parts ____

10. The matrix bed is composed of matrix cells which produce the:
    a) nail bed
    b) cuticle
    c) nail fold
    d) nail plate ____

11. The whitish moon shape under the nail plate is known as the:
    a) hyponychium
    b) nail fold
    c) lunula
    d) matrix ____

12. The most visible and functional part of the nail module is the:
    a) nail plate
    b) hyponychium
    c) cuticle
    d) onychodermal ____

13. The cuticle is also known as the:
    a) base of the nail
    b) lunula
    c) hyponychium
    d) eponychium
    _____

14. The "true cuticle" aids in:
    a) preventing injury and infection
    b) decreasing nail growth
    c) increasing nail growth
    d) none of the listed
    _____

15. A combination build-up of bed epithelium and hyponychial tissue is known as the:
    a) onychodermal band
    b) eponychium band
    c) hyponychium band
    d) lunula band
    _____

16. The nail bed and matrix bed is anchored to the underlying bone by the:
    a) muscles
    b) matrix
    c) specialized ligaments
    d) specialized tendons
    _____

17. The folds in the skin that forms the nail grooves are known as the:
    a) nail ligaments
    c) specialized ligaments
    c) nail folds
    d) onycholermal
    _____

18. The shape and thickness of the nail is determined by:
    a) the shape of the matrix bed
    b) the length of the matrix bed
    c) how fast it produces the nail plate
    d) a, b, and c
    _____

19. The nail plate is attached to the nail bed by a layer of tissue known as the:
    a) nail ligaments
    b) matrix layer
    c) bed epithelium
    d) bed folds
    _____

20. The main compound of the nail plate is fibrous protein called:
    a) phosphorus
    b) keratin
    c) calcium
    d) lunula
    _____

21. A nail disorder is a condition that can be caused by:
    a) an injury to the nail
    b) a disease in the body
    c) an imbalance in the body
    d) a, b, and c
    _____

22. A nail technician should never perform services on a client if there is evidence of:
    a) an infection
    b) ragged cuticles
    c) healthy skin
    d) a hangnail
    _____

23. Matrix bed problems are usually associated with:
    a) nail thickness
    b) nail coloring
    c) nail shapes
    d) dryness
    _____

24. Small white spots often seen under the surface of the nail plate are called:
    a) lunula
    b) leukonychia
    c) onychatrophia
    d) eponychium
    _____

25. Hangnails are caused by:
    a) dry cuticles
    b) nail biting
    c) polish
    d) buffing
    _____

26. The wasting away or atrophy of the nail is known as:
    a) onychauxis
    b) onychatrophia
    c) agnails
    d) leukonychia
    _____

27. The overgrowth of the nail is:
    a) onychauxis
    b) onychatrophia
    c) onychoophagy
    d) onychocryptosis _____

28. Nails, which are thin, white, and curved over the free edges are called:
    a) furrowed
    b) hangnails
    c) eggshell
    d) healthy _____

29. A black band seen under or within the nail plate extending from the proximal nail fold to the free edge is known as:
    a) furrows
    b) onychophagy
    c) infection
    d) melanonychia _____

30.) A condition in which a clot of blood forms under the nail plate due to injury to the nail bed is called a/an:
    a) bruised nail
    b) discolored nail
    c) infection
    d) inflammation _____

31. Long ridges that run lengthwise or across the nail are called:
    a) furrows
    b) onychophagy
    c) agnails
    d) leukonychia _____

32. Another term for an ingrown nail is:
    a) onychophagy
    b) furrows
    c) corrugations
    d) onychocyrptosis _____

33. Nails that have an increasing curvature throughout the nail plate are called:
    a) pincer nails
    b) tile nails
    c) eggshell nails
    d) plicatured nails _____

34. This condition develops as the nail reaches the end of the digit, and appears as a trumpet of cone formation:
    a) pincer nail
    b) tile-shaped nail
    c) eggshell nail
    d) bruised nail _____

35. When the surface of the nail is generally flat while one or both edges of the plate are folded at a 90-degree angle or move into the soft tissue nail margins, this is called a/an:
    a) trumpet nail
    b) pincer nail
    c) plicatured nail
    d) eggshell nail _____

36. The medical term for the nails that have been bitten enough to be deformed is called:
    a) oncychocryptosis
    b) onychophagy
    c) onychophosis
    d) pterygium _____

37. Split or brittle nails that have a series of lengthwise ridges are called:
    a) onychorrhexis
    b) onychophagy
    c) corrugations
    d) plicatured _____

38. Onychopathy or onychosis refers to a technical term for a:
    a) nail disease
    b) nail deformity
    c) nail shape
    d) nail injury _____

39. Abnormal scarring of the proximal or distal nail fold is called:
    a) pterygium
    b) plicatured
    c) corrugations
    d) agnails _____

40. Pseudomonas aeruginosa is a bacterium that can be found:
    a) in the soil and water   c) in the air
    b) in food   d) in the blood   ____

41. If a nail enhancement is not properly applied, pseudomonas bacteria can:
    a) infiltrate the lifted area   c) do nothing
    b) remain dormant   d) destroy the enhancement ____

42. If a client has mold present, no enhancements should be applied:
    a) for 2 months   c) for 3 weeks
    b) at any time   d) until there are no more
                                           visible signs of a problem ____

43. The number of fungi species that can cause infections to humans is:
    a) over 100,000   c) over 100
    b) less than 50   d) less than 25   ____

44. An injury to the nail that produces a portal of entry is prone to:
    a) a fungi infection   c) further injury
    b) becoming plicatured   d) becoming discolored   ____

45. Fungal infections occur more often on the:
    a) skin   c) toenails
    b) fingernails   d) hands   ____

46. A condition in which the nail loosens from the nail bed, usually beginning at the free edge and continuing to the lunula, is called:
    a) paronychia   c) onycholysis
    b) onychoptosis   d) onychomycosis   ____

47. An infection of the tissue around the nail is known as:
    a) onychoptosis   c) agnail
    b) paronychia   d) plicatured   ____

48. The shedding of the nail plate occurring in the fingernails and toenails is called:
    a) plicatured   c) onychomycosis
    b) paryonchia   d) onychomadesis   ____

49. Chronic paronychia is most often caused by:
    a) a virus   c) a yeast infection
    b) hereditary conditions   d) a bacterial infection   ____

50. A severe inflammation on the nail in which a lump of red tissue grows up from the nail bed to the nail plate is known as:
    a) paronychia   c) onychomadesis
    b) pyogenic granuloma   d) ventral pterygium   ____

THE SKIN AND ITS DISORDERS

1. The ability of healthy skin to regain its shape immediately after being pulled away from the bone is called:
   a) electricity
   b) elasticity
   c) stimuli
   d) fluidity ____

2. The skin performs all of these jobs for the body except:
   a) protection
   b) heat regulation
   c) nutrition
   d) excretion ____

3. The outer layer of skin is called the:
   a) dermis
   b) epidermis
   c) papillary layer
   d) subcutaneous tissue ____

4. The deepest layer of skin is called the:
   a) dermis
   b) epidermis
   c) papilla
   d) subcutaneous layer ____

5. The epidermis contains no:
   a) nerves
   b) keratin
   c) blood vessels
   d) cells ____

6. This layer of the skin is composed of dead epithelial cells that have become keratinized:
   a) stratum lucidum
   b) stratum granulosum
   c) melanin
   d) stratum coerneum ____

7. The small epidermal layer composed of clear cells is the:
   a) stratum corneum
   b) stratum lucidum
   c) stratum granulosum
   d) melanin ____

8. Cells that look like granules are in the layer of epidermis called:
   a) stratum lucidum
   b) stratum corneum
   c) stratum granulosum
   d) basal layer ____

9. Melanin is found in this epidermis layer:
   a) stratum lucidum
   b) basal layer
   c) stratum corneum
   d) stratum granulosum ____

10. Blood vessels and nerves are found in the:
    a) dermis
    b) epidermis
    c) follicle
    d) stratum corneum ____

11. The dermal layer which lies directly under the epidermis is the:
    a) adipose tissue
    b) papillary layer
    c) tactile corpuscles
    d) horny layer ____

12. Fat cells, blood vessels, and sweat glands are found in the:
    a) subcutaneous layer
    b) papillae
    c) epidermis
    d) reticular layer ____

13. The fatty tissue found in the subcutaneous layer of the dermis is called:
   a) energy cells
   b) cellulite
   c) adipose
   d) sebum
   _____

14. Arrector pili muscles can cause:
   a) spasms
   b) arthritis
   c) hair growth
   d) goose bumps
   _____

15. Sensory nerve endings are most abundant in the:
   a) toes
   b) fingertips and soles of the feet
   c) nose
   d) eyes
   _____

16. The common name for the sudoriferous glands is:
   a) oil glands
   b) hormones
   c) sweat glands
   d) lymph nodes
   _____

17. The small opening in the skin surface through which the sudoriferous glands eliminate waste is the:
   a) papilla
   b) sweat pore
   c) hair shaft
   d) secretory nerve
   _____

18. A structural change in tissue caused by injury and disease is called a:
   a) lesion
   b) pustule
   c) fissure
   d) scar
   _____

19. A semi-solid or fluid lump above and below the skin surface is called a:
   a) papule
   b) macule
   c) cyst
   d) bulla
   _____

20. A lump on the skin with an inflamed base and a head containing pus is called a:
   a) tubercle
   b) pustule
   c) scale
   d) scar
   _____

21. Severe dandruff is an example of:
   a) scales
   b) crust
   c) fissure
   d) bulla
   _____

22. A chronic inflammatory skin disorder characterized by itching, burning, formations of scales, and oozing blisters of unknown origin is known as:
   a) eczema
   b) dandruff
   c) psoriasis
   d) herpes simplex
   _____

23. A generalized disease that may produce mild to severe effects on the skin is called:
   a) eczema
   b) psoriasis
   c) dandruff
   d) herpes simplex
   _____

24. If a client has had any form of psoriasis, it is suggested that before beginning a service you consult your client's:
   a) doctor
   b) pharmacist
   c) social worker
   d) dentist
   _____

25. A localized reaction of the skin to friction from an external source is known as:
   a) fever blister
   b) friction blister
   c) eczema
   d) psoriasis
   _____

26. An enlarged area of irritated skin with its edges blending onto the normal surrounding skin is called a:
a) blister
b) bump
c) verruca
d) callus
_____

27. Warts are caused by:
a) a parasite
b) skin deterioration
c) a viral infection
d) a bacterial infection
_____

28. Warts rarely occur in:
a) children under 7
b) children under 5
c) teenagers
d) young adults
_____

29. Warts are most commonly seen on the:
a) feet and hands
b) back
c) knees and elbows
d) neck and shoulders
_____

30. The probability of a nail technician contracting a wart virus is:
a) less than 20%
b) less than 10%
c) less than 50%
d) not possible at all
_____

31. Yeast and mold fall into the classification of:
a) virus
b) bacteria
c) infection
d) fungi
_____

32. Fungal infections of the skin can be caused by:
a) an infected pet
b) soil
c) contact with an infected person
d) a, b, and c
_____

33. A fungal infection characterized by blisters that may break, ooze, and itch, and may cause the skin to crack is the kind called:
a) acute inflammatory
b) mild inflammatory
c) chronic inflammatory
d) chronic hyperkeratotic
_____

34. When the skin becomes whitish and has painful fissures develop between the toes, this is a typical example of tinea pedis or:
a) tinea capitis
b) athlete's foot
c) hyperkeratotic
d) plantar warts
_____

35. The most common "tumor" of the skin is the:
a) pigmented nevus
b) tinea capitis
c) herpes simplex
d) melanoma
_____

36. If a client has an acute inflammatory form of a fungal infection, the nail technician:
a) may perform services
b) may not perform services
c) may perform services while wearing gloves
d) may apply antiseptic to the area and perform services
_____

37. This percentage of cancers diagnosed in the U.S. is melanoma:
a) 10%
b) 20%
c) 1%
d) 5%
_____

38. A skin infection common in dental staff and others involved with the care of the mouth is:
a) tinea capitis
b) melanoma
c) amelamotic
d) herpes simplex
_____

39. A congenital absence of melanin pigment in the body is known as:
    a) albinism
    b) keratoma
    c) lentigine
    d) vitiligo
    _____

40. Liver spots are also called:
    a) lentigines
    b) chloasma
    c) albinism
    d) nevus
    _____

41. Another name for freckles is:
    a) tan
    b) chloasma
    c) lentigines
    d) nevus
    _____

42. An acquired form of leucoderma that affects the skin and hair is:
    a) melanoma
    b) lentigines
    c) vitiligo
    d) pigmented nevus
    _____

chapter 9

CLIENT CONSULTATION

1. A conversation you have with a client before starting the service is called:
   - a) chat
   - b) consultation
   - c) service recording
   - d) conduct
   ____

2. During a consultation you need to assess all of the following aspects except the:
   - a) client's health
   - b) client's skin
   - c) client's lifestyle
   - d) client's hairstyle
   ____

3. The analysis and recommendations are two parts of a client:
   - a) service
   - b) manicure
   - c) consultation
   - d) procedure
   ____

4. The safety of your client will depend upon your:
   - a) knowledge
   - b) questions
   - c) observations
   - d) a, b, and c
   ____

5. During this section you ask questions and look closely at the client's skin and nails:
   - a) recommendation section
   - b) analysis section
   - c) greeting section
   - d) procedure section
   ____

6. Recommendations are made after:
   - a) the client's goals are defined
   - b) the analysis is performed
   - c) you have made visual observations
   - d) a, b, and c
   ____

7. Home care recommendations are suggested to:
   - a) make more money
   - b) impress your co-workers
   - c) aid the client
   - d) impress your boss
   ____

8. Your first opportunity to portray yourself as a professional to your client is:
   - a) during your service
   - b) after your service
   - c) during your consultation
   - d) before your consultation
   ____

9. A professional consultation technique includes all of the following except:
   - a) being friendly
   - b) focusing on your client
   - c) supporting your recommendations
   - d) talking to co-workers during your consultation
   ____

10. The difference between being a professional and just "doing nails" is:
    a) a well-done consultation
    b) not using sanitation procedures
    c) not being prepared
    d) having a good hairstyle

    ____

11. You should think of your recommendations as:
    a) educating your clients
    b) impressing your boss
    c) selling more products
    d) making more money

    ____

12. Your client's health/record card should be kept in:
    a) your table drawer
    b) a drawer at your home
    c) a convenient location for every nail tech
    d) the dispensary

    ____

13. The type of information usually found on a client health/record card includes all of the following except the:
    a) client's name
    b) client's address
    c) client's phone number
    d) client's social security number

    ____

14. Information about your client's general health should be found in the:
    a) general section
    b) medical section
    c) client's profile
    d) service section

    ____

15. An entry should be made on the client's record card:
    a) every time they receive a service
    b) every 2 weeks
    c) whenever you have time to complete the card
    d) when you think about it

    ____

16. When a client's record/health card is maintained adequately, this shows your client:
    a) that you are professional
    b) that you care about their safety
    c) that you care about their health
    d) a, b, and c

    ____

17. Knowing about a client's general health will indicate the safeness of performing a:
    a) basic manicure
    b) basic pedicure
    c) hand or foot massage
    d) artificial nail removal

    ____

18. When a client's nail technician is not available, the client can be serviced by referring to the:
    a) client's hairstylist
    b) salon that previously serviced them
    c) owner's instructions
    d) client's service record

    ____

MANICURING

Chapter 10

1. The number of types of nail technology tools is:
   a) three
   b) four
   c) five
   d) six _____

2. Permanent tools used in nail technology are called:
   a) implements
   b) overhead
   c) equipment
   d) materials _____

3. The lamp on a manicure table should have a bulb with a wattage of:
   a) 40
   b) 50
   c) 60
   d) 100 _____

4. A low wattage bulb is not adequate to:
   a) produce sufficient light
   b) dry polish
   c) warm the client's nails
   d) kill germs _____

5. A high wattage bulb will interfere with products when performing:
   a) sculptured nails
   b) pedicures
   c) wet sanitizing
   d) hand massage _____

6. A fingerbowl is used to soak the client's fingers in warm water and:
   a) disinfectant
   b) dish detergent
   c) alcohol
   d) antibacterial soap _____

7. A client cushion can be fashioned by the technician from a:
   a) pillow
   b) towel
   c) foam square
   d) cotton coil _____

8. Implements include all the following except a/an:
   a) electric nail dryer
   b) orangewood stick
   c) steel pusher
   d) metal nail file _____

9. Emery boards, orangewood sticks, and cotton are items that are:
   a) reusable
   b) sterile
   c) disposable
   d) expensive _____

10. The common name for a steel pusher is:
    a) cuticle nipper
    b) cuticle pusher
    c) orangewood stick
    d) emery board _____

11. The coarse side of an emery board is used to:
    a) shape the free edge
    b) bevel the nail
    c) file the top of the nail
    d) etch the natural nail _____

12. A good choice for filing soft or fragile nails is a/an:
    a) metal nail file
    b) chamois buffer
    c) fingernail clipper
    d) emery board _____

13. To lift small bits of cuticle from the nail, use:
    a) cuticle nipper
    b) tweezers
    c) an orangewood stick
    d) a cotton ball _____

14. It is not a good idea to save an emery board in a plastic bag for each client, due to the growth of:
a) papules
b) fungus
c) bacteria
d) parasites ____

15. To add shine to the nail and smooth out wavy ridges, you should use a/an:
a) metal nail file
b) emery board
c) nail brush
d) chamois buffer ____

16. To cut filing time on long nails, shorten nails with a:
a) cuticle nipper
b) fingernail clipper
c) nail buffer
d) metal nail file ____

17. Materials are single-use supplies that are used during a manicure and include all the following except:
a) cotton balls
b) towels
c) plastic bags
d) nail brush ____

18. A nail strengthener is applied to the natural nail:
a) before the base coat
b) after the base coat
c) after nail polish
d) after the top coat ____

19. Nail cosmetics include all of the following except:
a) top coat
b) base coat
c) alcohol
d) cuticle oil ____

20. The basic nail shapes include all of the following except:
a) square
b) hexagonal
c) round
d) oval ____

21. The best nail shape for clients who work on typewriters, computers, and assembly lines is:
a) squoval
b) round
c) oval
d) pointed ____

22. The most common nail shape for male clients is:
a) square
b) round
c) oval
d) pointed ____

23. The best nail shape choice for businesswomen is often:
a) square
b) round
c) oval
d) pointed ____

24. If you accidentally nick your client during a manicure and blood becomes present, the first thing you should do is:
a) have the client wash his or her hands
b) put on gloves
c) apply an antiseptic
d) tell your boss ____

25. As a professional nail technician, all services you perform will have three parts:
a) pre-service, manicure, post-service
b) consultation, procedure, retail sale
c) pre-service, pedicure, retail sale
d) pre-service, procedure, post-service ____

26. To reduce heat during buffing, spray the client's nails with:
a) hairspray
b) water
c) alcohol
d) oil ____

27. To mix polish, you should:
a) shake the bottle
b) tap the bottle on a table
c) stir the polish with a brush
d) roll the bottle between your palms ____

28. When the entire nail plate is polished, the application is called:
a) slimline
b) lunula
c) full coverage
d) hairline tip ____

29. The French Manicure is a great base for:
a) pale polish
b) buffing
c) nail art
d) artificial tips ____

30. Clients with ridged and brittle nails or dry cuticles should benefit from:
a) a reconditioning hot oil manicure
b) a French Manicure
c) gentle scrubbing
d) gel nails ____

31. Most men generally need more work done on their:
a) free edge
b) hangnails
c) buffing
d) cuticles ____

32. Paraffin treatments can be given to clients with:
a) freckles
b) eczema
c) rashes
d) swollen veins ____

33. You should never use an electric file on a client:
a) in a salon
b) in a school
c) until you have been taught and have practiced
d) who has arthritis ____

34. Paraffin wax treatments work by trapping heat and moisture in and:
a) closing the pores of the skin
b) sanitizing the skin
c) cooling the skin
d) opening the pores of the skin ____

35. The temperature of paraffin wax is generally maintained between:
a) 100-110 degrees Fahrenheit
b) 100-110 degrees Celsius
c) 125-130 degrees Celsius
d) 125-130 degrees Fahrenheit ____

36. Effleurage is a massage movement that consists of:
a) light stroking
b) kneading
c) wringing
d) rotating the elbow ____

37. The massage service should not be performed on a client with any of the following conditions except:
a) high blood pressure
b) muscle aches
c) stroke
d) heart condition ____

38. Vigorous massage of joints can be painful for clients with:
a) hangnails
b) dry skin
c) arthritis
d) a lung condition ____

39. Spa manicures encompasses extensive knowledge of nail care as well as:
a) skin care
b) hair care
c) massage techniques
d) pedicuring ____

40. Additional techniques that can be included into a spa manicure may be:
a) aromatherapy
b) hand masks
c) reflexology
d) a, b, and c ____

PEDICURING

1. Trimming, shaping, and polishing toenails as well as performing a foot massage is called:
   a) manicuring
   b) toe trimming
   c) podiatry
   d) pedicuring ____

2. When taking an appointment for a pedicure, inform the client polish will not smear if they:
   a) wear open-toed shoes/sandals
   b) wear cotton socks
   c) wear black hose
   d) wear pumps ____

3. The pedicuring station includes all the following except a:
   a) client chair
   b) telephone
   c) client footrest
   d) technician's chair ____

4. When handling the foot during a pedicure, you should be firm and:
   a) light
   b) gentle
   c) irregular
   d) rough ____

5. To remove dry skin or callus growths, use a/an:
   a) foot file
   b) antibacterial soap
   c) antiseptic spray
   d) antifungal agent ____

6. An antiseptic spray for pedicuring contains:
   a) talcum powder
   b) an antifungal agent
   c) an antibacterial soap
   d) foot lotion ____

7. During the pedicure procedure, the client's feet should be placed on a:
   a) toe separator
   b) dry floor
   c) clean terry towel
   d) pedicure slipper ____

8. You may not perform a pedicure on a client with any of the following conditions except:
   a) athlete's foot
   b) fungus
   c) infection
   d) hang nail ____

9. When water is spilled during pedicuring, wipe it up immediately to prevent:
   a) falls
   b) bacteria growth
   c) fungus growth
   d) athlete's foot ____

10. The purpose of soaking the feet prior to the pedicure procedure is:
    a) to remove calluses
    b) sanitation
    c) to soften hangnails
    d) to relax the client ____

11. Toe separators should be inserted before this pedicure step:
    a) clipping nails
    b) removing polish
    c) brushing nails
    d) filing nails ____

12. Toenails should be filed straight across, with corners:
    a) straight
    b) square
    c) slightly rounded
    d) filed into ____

13. Cuticle solvent may be used to soften excess skin below the nail's:
    a) free edge
    b) bed
    c) polish
    d) root ____

14. Most pedicure services are performed by starting with the:
    a) left foot, little toe
    b) right foot, little toe
    c) left foot, big toe
    d) right foot, big toe ____

15. After massaging the foot and before applying polish, you must:
    a) remove all lotion from the toenails
    b) rinse the feet
    c) apply cuticle remover
    d) powder the feet ____

16. To avoid smearing polish, the top coat should be followed by:
    a) a second top coat
    b) instant nail dry
    c) warm, blowing air
    d) cool, blowing air ____

17. The three basic forms of hand manipulations utilized in therapeutic massage include effleurage, petrissage, and:
    a) vibration
    b) squeezing
    c) friction
    d) tapotment ____

18. To maintain the pedicure at home, the client should purchase all the following products except:
    a) polish
    b) antibacterial soap
    c) lotion
    d) top coat ____

19. Following a pedicure service, basins, tables, and footrests should be sanitized with:
    a) steam
    b) dry heat
    c) a hospital-grade disinfectant
    d) fungicide ____

20. Before use on a client, pedicure implements must be sanitized for at least:
    a) 5 minutes
    b) 20 minutes
    c) 30 minutes
    d) 60 minutes ____

21. Between each service, your table should be arranged for:
    a) basic set-up
    b) best appearance
    c) proper sanitation
    d) clean top ____

22. The client with high blood pressure, heart condition or stroke should not have a massage without permission from a:
    a) chiropractor
    b) spouse
    c) salon owner
    d) physician ____

23. The foot massage begins with:
    a) joint relaxer movements
    b) effleurage on top
    c) effleurage on heel
    d) metatarsal scissors ____

24. Clients will find effleurage:
    a) painful to joints
    b) stimulating
    c) relaxing
    d) to cause burning sensation ____

25. To perform joint movement for toes, toes are moved so as to create a:
    a) popping sound
    b) figure eight
    c) complete circle
    d) square ____

26. Nail rasps are used to:
    a) shape the free edge
    b) remove debris from the nail margins
    c) thin the toenails
    d) smooth the nail edges in the grooves ____

27. You should inquire as to whether a massage should be performed if the client:
    a) has had foot surgery
    b) has ingrown toenails
    c) has dry cuticles
    d) has a verruca ____

28. Flexibility is promoted by this technique:
    a) thumb compression
    b) effleurage
    c) metatarsal scissors
    d) fist twist ____

29. Fist twist compression is a friction movement which requires:
    a) great concentration
    b) deep rubbing
    c) gentleness
    d) many applications ____

30. The tapotement movements used to end a massage are commonly known as:
    a) final effleurage
    b) tapping touches
    c) tingle toes
    d) percussion movements ____

31. Basic product classes for pedicure services include soaks, massage products, and:
    a) reflexology
    b) scrubs
    c) aromatherapy
    d) a, b, and c ____

32. Sea salts contribute to:
    a) dehydration of the skin
    b) super dehydration of the skin
    c) super hydration of the skin
    d) minimal hydration of the skin ____

33. To aid in removing dry flaky skin and calluses, which build up on the foot, use:
    a) massage products
    b) soaks
    c) scrubs
    d) aromatherapy oils ____

34. Massage preparations are used to lubricate, moisturize, and:
    a) invigorate the skin
    b) decrease circulation
    c) remove skin build-up
    d) exfoliate dead skin ____

35. Add-on products are products offered to enhance or:
    a) raise the cost of the pedicure
    b) expedite the pedicure
    c) slow down the pedicure
    d) lower the cost of the pedicure ____

36. Clients with impaired circulation, loss of feeling, or other diabetic related problems should not receive:
    a) soaks
    b) aromatherapy treatments
    c) hot wax treatments
    d) a polish application ____

37. A major advantage of a diamond nail file is that it:
    a) is inexpensive
    b) can be given to the client for home care
    c) is disposable after use
    d) can be easily sanitized ____

ELECTRIC FILING

chapter 12

1. The AEFM was formed to establish the standards of electric filing in:
   a) 1996
   b) 1997
   c) 1986
   d) 1998 ____

2. Do electric files damage the nails?
   a) no, if properly used
   b) yes, always to some extent
   c) most of the time
   d) never ____

3. Common ways to cause nail damage are by Rings of fire and:
   a) practicing
   b) heat
   c) bands of fire
   d) cold ____

4. Heat during electric filing is caused by:
   a) too little friction
   b) too much pressure
   c) too little pressure
   d) no friction ____

5. The bit made from natural materials that must be disposed of between clients is the:
   a) buffing bit
   b) pedicure bit
   c) natural nail bit
   d) carbide bit ____

6. The most commonly used file in the nail industry is the:
   a) cable-driven type
   b) micromotor type
   c) belt-driven type
   d) battery-driven type ____

7. An electric file is used for saving time and:
   a) skills
   b) practice
   c) money
   d) energy ____

8. RPM stands for:
   a) Repellent Power Motor
   b) Rotating Per Minute
   c) Revolutions Per Minute
   d) Rotary Power Movement ____

9. If a bit is rotating at 5,000 RPM, this means that the bit is hitting the nail:
   a) 5,000 times per minute
   b) 5,000 times every 5 minutes
   c) 5,000 times every 10 minutes
   d) 5,000 times in one hour ____

10. The average nail tech uses a machine that has:
    a) 1,000-2,000 RPM
    b) 5,000-15,000 RPM
    c) 1,000-30,000 RPM
    d) none of the listed ____

11. The amount of resistance in the electric file as the bit turns is called the:
    a) torque
    b) residual resistance
    c) RPM
    d) turning resistance ____

12. A perfectly balanced bit is called:
    a) concentric
    b) torque
    c) a diamond bit
    d) a barrel ____

13. When using an electric filing machine you should:
    a) wipe the bit with a cloth before reusing
    b) give the bit to your client after using
    c) never use the same bit on every client without disinfecting
    d) change the bit after every two clients ____

14. The bit should always be placed on the nail:
    a) at a 10° angle
    b) at a 35° angle
    c) at a 45° angle
    d) flat ____

15. Ridges that are created when using the bit at the wrong angle at the cuticle area are called:
    a) friction ridges
    b) pressure ridges
    c) Rings of fire
    d) Rings of pressure ____

16. Pressure causes friction, and friction causes:
    a) mold
    b) bumps
    c) heat
    d) cold ____

17. For prepping the natural nail and removing the shine, it is recommended to use:
    a) a synthetic natural nail bit
    b) a diamond nail bit
    c) a sanding bit
    d) a metal bit ____

18. The use of buffing creams:
    a) should be avoided
    b) will enhance the shine power
    c) should be restricted to natural nails only
    d) do nothing for the nail's shine ____

19. If the electric file is causing your client discomfort, you should:
    a) slow down the RPM
    b) use less pressure
    c) practice more
    d) do all the listed ____

20. A sign that you might be working too fast and applying too much pressure will be:
    a) the bit grabs and wraps around the finger
    b) the machine smokes
    c) the bit stops working
    d) the nail feels cool ____

21. Speed and safety while using an electric drill comes from:
    a) observing educational videos
    b) going to educational shows
    c) actual practicing
    d) a, b, and c ____

chapter 13

AROMATHERAPY

1. The literal translation of aromatherapy means:
   a) therapy through aroma
   b) treatments through aroma
   c) aroma treatments
   d) air freshener
   ____

2. Oils that have been extracted by various forms of distillation from botanical sources in various parts of a plant are known as:
   a) plant oils
   b) botanical oils
   c) flower oils
   d) essential oils
   ____

3. Essential oils are beneficial in all of the following except:
   a) manicures
   b) pedicures
   c) facials
   d) cooking
   ____

4. This oil is beneficial in overall first aid and is antiviral and antibacterial:
   a) chamomile
   b) rosemary
   c) lavender
   d) orange
   ____

5. This oil is suggested to aid digestion and sooth the nerves:
   a) orange
   b) chamomile
   c) lavender
   d) rosemary
   ____

6. This oil is suggested for stimulating circulation, relieving pain and decongestion:
   a) neroli
   b) rosemary
   c) cypress
   d) vanilla
   ____

7. This oil clears sinuses, is an antiseptic, decongestant, and stimulus:
   a) peppermint
   b) cypress
   c) tea tree oil
   d) bergamot
   ____

8. A base oil to which the essential oil is added is known as:
   a) secondary oil
   b) carrier oil
   c) direct oil additive
   d) primary oil
   ____

9. You should always perform a patch test before using oil:
   a) in a diffuser
   b) to add aroma to the air
   c) directly to the skin
   d) on the hair
   ____

10. The oil that resembles our bodies' sebum is:
    a) grapeseed oil
    b) avocado oil
    c) sweet almond oil
    d) jojoba oil
    ____

11. In the foot there are actually more than:
    a) 50,000 nerve endings
    b) 10,000 nerve endings
    c) 5,000 nerve endings
    d) 2,000 nerve endings
    ____

12. For spring and summer you should use:
    a) light oils
    b) heavier oils
    c) medium weight oils
    d) a mixture of oils
    ____

13. For fall and winter you should use:
    a) light oils
    b) heavier oils
    c) medium-weight oils
    d) a mixture of oils
    ____

14. Essential oils for beauty services should be purchased from:
    a) a hospital
    b) a discount store
    c) the beauty industry
    d) a drug store ____

15. If a woman is pregnant you should not use:
    a) lemon
    b) grapeseed
    c) lavender
    d) peppermint ____

chapter 14

NAIL TIPS

1. A nail tip is an artificial nail made of any of the following, except:
   a) plastic
   b) rubber
   c) nylon
   d) acetate
   ____

2. Tips are applied to the natural nail to give the client's nails added:
   a) strength
   b) wells
   c) length
   d) buffers
   ____

3. A tip with no overlay is very:
   a) beautiful
   b) weak
   c) strong
   d) finished-looking
   ____

4. A tip with no overlay is considered a/an:
   a) temporary service
   b) finished nail
   c) unfinished nail
   d) natural look
   ____

5. To smooth the natural nail and remove the shine, you should use an:
   a) adhesive
   b) antibacterial agent
   c) alcohol sanitizer
   d) abrasive
   ____

6. The point of contact for the artificial nail tip and the natural nail plate is called the:
   a) extension
   b) glue
   c) well
   d) bed
   ____

7. Tip wells are full or:
   a) quarter
   b) partial
   c) three-quarters
   d) three-eighths
   ____

8. The artificial nail tip should never cover more than this amount of the natural nail plate:
   a) $1/2$
   b) $1/3$
   c) $1/4$
   d) $1/5$
   ____

9. Before receiving a nail tip application, the client should wash her hands with:
   a) alcohol
   b) antibacterial soap
   c) fungicide
   d) lanolin
   ____

10. Buff the nail plate to remove:
    a) soap residue
    b) nail polish
    c) dust
    d) natural oil
    ____

11. Properly sized tips will cover the nail plate from:
    a) the lunula to the free edge
    b) sidewall to sidewall
    c) the lunula to mid-nail
    d) the free edge out
    ____

12. Nail tip procedures are performed starting with the:
    a) little finger, right hand
    b) thumb, left hand
    c) little finger, left hand
    d) thumb, right hand
    ____

13. Adhesive should be applied:
    a) from the free edge to 1/16" away from the cuticle area
    b) to the entire nail plate
    c) from the cuticle area to the middle of the nail
    d) from the middle of the nail plate to the free edge ____

14. Adhesive is applied to the:
    a) nail plate
    b) lunula
    c) cuticle area
    d) free edge ____

15. To help prevent trapped air bubbles in adhesive, the adhesive may be applied to the:
    a) free edge of tip
    b) sidewall
    c) well of the tip
    d) spatula ____

16. When sliding on tips, stop against the free edge at a:
    a) 33° angle
    b) 45° angle
    c) 50° angle
    d) 55° angle ____

17. Hold the tip in place until dry for approximately:
    a) 3 to 4 seconds
    b) 5 to 10 seconds
    c) 12 to 15 seconds
    d) 15 to 20 seconds ____

18. A bead of adhesive is applied to the seam between the natural nail plate and the tip to:
    a) add beauty
    b) strengthen stress points
    c) add length
    d) smooth ridges ____

19. Artificial nail tips should not be trimmed straight across, as this will cause the plastic to:
    a) weaken
    b) lift
    c) crack
    d) break ____

20. To blend the artificial tip with the natural nail, you should:
    a) use extra adhesive
    b) use trimmers
    c) gently file and buff
    d) cover the nail with a tip ____

21. A tip should blend with the natural nail so there is no:
    a) air bubble
    b) excess adhesive
    c) jagged edge
    d) visible line ____

22. A nail tip should be covered with:
    a) wrap, acrylic, or a gel nail
    b) two base coats
    c) three polish coats
    d) nail strengthener and base coat ____

23. Clients who want temporary tips need a:
    a) quick manicure
    b) two-appointment service
    c) three-appointment service
    d) four-appointment service ____

24. Clients wearing tips need to come back to the salon for service:
    a) weekly
    b) monthly
    c) biannually
    d) yearly ____

25. Using the tip well cutting application, the well of the tip is:
    a) split
    b) notched
    c) removed completely
    d) cut 1/4 inch off ____

26. During weekly maintenance, tips should be:
    a) clipped shorter
    b) removed and reapplied
    c) reglued at seam
    d) sanitized _____

27. To remove polish on nail tips, use a/an:
    a) acetone remover
    b) buffer block
    c) cuticle remover
    d) non-acetone remover _____

28. Never nip off artificial nail tips, as you might cause damage to the:
    a) natural free edge
    b) nail root
    c) nail bed
    d) cuticle _____

29. To remove artificial nail tips, use glue remover or:
    a) a buffer block
    b) acetone
    c) an emery board
    d) a steel pusher _____

30. After soaking in remover, softened tips are carefully removed using a/an:
    a) steel pusher
    b) emery board
    c) nail clipper
    d) orangewood stick _____

31. To remove glue residue from a natural nail, use a/an:
    a) fine buffer block
    b) cuticle oil
    c) orangewood stick
    d) cuticle remover _____

NAIL WRAPS

chapter 15

1. Nail wraps consist of nail-size pieces of cloth bonded to:
   a) the underside of the free edge
   b) the top of the nail
   c) the sides of the nail
   d) the top of the free edge only
   _____

2. Nail wraps are used on natural nails or artificial tips to:
   a) provide a base for polish
   b) hide poor technical work
   c) repair or strengthen
   d) provide a base for nail art
   _____

3. Fabric wraps are made from all of the following material except:
   a) fiberglass
   b) cotton
   c) linen
   d) silk
   _____

4. When adhesive is applied to a silk wrap, the wrap becomes:
   a) strong
   b) smooth
   c) wrinkled
   d) transparent
   _____

5. The linen wrap must be covered with colored polish because it is:
   a) closely woven
   b) opaque
   c) heavy
   d) transparent
   _____

6. Polish remover causes paper wraps to:
   a) rip
   b) become brittle
   c) dissolve
   d) turn yellow
   _____

7. The pointed applicator tip on nail adhesive is called a/an:
   a) extender tip
   b) bonding tip
   c) spatula tip
   d) cuticle tip
   _____

8. Nail wrap procedures begin on the:
   a) little finger, right hand
   b) thumb, right hand
   c) little finger, left hand
   d) thumb, left hand
   _____

9. The adhesive is applied to all ten nails on the:
   a) free edge
   b) entire surface
   c) lunula
   d) sidewall
   _____

10. The fabric should be cut to:
    a) 1/2 the size of the nail plate
    b) 1/4 the size of the nail plate
    c) the length of the nail plate or tip
    d) the width or shape of the nail plate or tip
    _____

11. The final two adhesive applications in a fabric wrap are applied:
    a) over fabric
    b) under fabric
    c) to the cuticle
    d) 10 minutes apart
    _____

12. To clean adhesive extender tips, soak in acetone and then clear the hole with a clean:
    a) cotton swab
    b) pipe cleaner
    c) orangewood stick
    d) toothpick
    _____

13. To acquaint clients with the latest manicure looks, host:
    a) manicure lessons   c) a nail fashion night
    b) a cosmetics party   d) a fund-raiser event   ____

14. Offer clients a nailcare fashion kit with a gift certificate and:
    a) nail polish   c) hand cream
    b) trial-sized products   d) emery boards   ____

15. Fabric wraps are maintained after two weeks with a:
    a) glue fill   c) water manicure
    b) polish change   d) fabric fill   ____

16. In a glue fill, adhesive is applied first to the:
    a) free edge   c) new nail growth
    b) entire nail   d) edges of the nail wrap   ____

17. A purpose of applying adhesive to the entire nail in a glue fill
    is to:
    a) smooth the ridges   c) apply a new wrap
    b) reseal the wrap   d) form a base for polish   ____

18. In a four week fabric wrap maintenance visit, the new nail
    growth is:
    a) covered with fabric   c) ignored
    b) polished   d) measured   ____

19. A strip of fabric cut to 1/8 inch is called a:
    a) repair patch   c) center application
    b) fabric wrap   d) stress strip   ____

20. A piece of fabric cut to completely cover a crack or break in the
    nail is called a:
    a) repair patch   c) complete application
    b) fabric wrap   d) stress strip   ____

21. The lightweight tissue paper used in wraps is called:
    a) wrapping paper   c) liquid paper
    b) mending tissue   d) onionskin   ____

22. The heavy adhesive used in paper wraps is called:
    a) paste   c) liquid nails
    b) glue   d) mending liquid   ____

23. Paper wraps are used to give a nail:
    a) length   c) strength
    b) regrowth area   d) a base for nail art   ____

24. Paper wraps are not recommended for nails which are:
    a) short   c) pointed
    b) extra long   d) square   ____

25. When fitting the tissue, the edges should be:
    a) feathered   c) curved
    b) straight   d) past the sidewall   ____

26. In applying a paper wrap, the mending tissue should be tucked:
    a) around the sidewall   c) under the free edge
    b) at the nail plate center   d) at the lunula   ____

27. After smoothing the applied tissue, the top and free edges of the nail should be covered with two or three coats of:
    a) mending liquid
    b) acrylic
    c) base coat
    d) top coat ____

28. Before applying polish, the paper wrap's surface should be smoothed by applying:
    a) base coat
    b) ridge filler
    c) mending liquid
    d) buffing compound ____

29. A polish made up of tiny fibers to strengthen and preserve the natural nail is:
    a) nail strengthener
    b) base coat
    c) liquid nail wrap
    d) top coat ____

30. Liquid nail wrap is applied to the nail by:
    a) spray
    b) spatula
    c) soaking in it
    d) brush ____

chapter 16

ACRYLIC NAILS

1. Acrylic nails are also known as:
   a) nail tips
   b) sculptured nails
   c) plastic nails
   d) hard nails ____

2. Sculptured nails are created by combining acrylic liquid with:
   a) paper wrap
   b) acrylic powder
   c) silk wrap
   d) fiberglass ____

3. The acrylic liquid is known as the:
   a) polymer
   b) monomer
   c) reactive agent
   d) residual agent ____

4. The acrylic powder is known as the:
   a) polymer
   b) monomer
   c) reactive agent
   d) residual agent ____

5. When the reaction completes its process it is called a:
   a) catalyst
   b) monomer
   c) polymer
   d) reactor ____

6. Special additives are blended into the liquids to:
   a) ensure color stabilization
   b) given strength and flexibility
   c) prevent the liquid from hardening
   d) a, b, and c ____

7. The helper that brings the polymer and monomer together as a whole is known as the:
   a) additive
   b) reactor
   c) catalyst
   d) agent ____

8. When the catalyst comes in contact with the monomer:
   a) heat is developed
   b) cold is developed
   c) nothing happens
   d) a dehydrator is developed ____

9. The heat from the catalytic reaction starts a chain of movements transferring heat from:
   a) one monomer bead to another
   b) one polymer bead to another
   c) one reactor bead to another
   d) one catalysis bead to another ____

10. The process that continues to transfer until the last polymer bead receives heat is known as:
    a) monomerization
    b) polymerization
    c) catalysis
    d) priming ____

11. To clean and remove moisture on the nail plate you apply:
    a) an antiseptic
    b) primer
    c) a dehydrator
    d) sanitizer ____

12. To enhance the adhesion of the acrylic to the natural nail, apply:
    a) an antiseptic   c) a dehydrator
    b) primer   d) sanitizer   ____

13. Small containers of glue should be purchased because:
    a) they cost less   c) they only have a
    b) they take up less space   6-month shelf life
        d) they are easier to handle and use   ____

14. Unused monomer should not be poured back into the original container because:
    a) it is contaminated after use   c) it has polymerized
    b) it has lost its strength   d) it has already had a reaction   ____

15. The best brush for acrylic application is made from:
    a) synthetic hair   c) sable hair
    b) yak hair   d) camel hair   ____

16. Safety glasses and gloves should always be worn when applying:
    a) dehydrator   c) polymer
    b) monomer   d) primer   ____

17. The nail form should be positioned so that it fits snugly, and the natural nail free edge is:
    a) under the form   c) $1/16$ inch away
    b) butted to form the edge   d) over the form   ____

18. Primer should dry on nails until the color is:
    a) yellow   c) pink
    b) chalky white   d) pale blue   ____

19. To form an acrylic ball, the sable brush is dipped into:
    a) liquid, then powder   c) powder, liquid, powder
    b) powder, then liquid   d) liquid, powder, liquid   ____

20. Touching the primed area of the nail with a wet brush prior to acrylic application will cause the acrylic to:
    a) remain liquid   c) separate
    b) harden rapidly   d) lift   ____

21. In acrylic application, the first acrylic ball is used to form the:
    a) nail plate   c) entire nail
    b) free edge   d) sidewalls   ____

22. Acrylic should be applied by using this brush technique:
    a) dab and press   c) "x"-pattern
    b) paint stroke   d) dot, then paint   ____

23. For a natural-looking nail, acrylic application near the cuticle, sidewall, and free edge should be:
    a) $1/16$ inch away   c) extremely thin
    b) moderately thick   d) white powder   ____

24. Acrylic nails are dry when gentle tapping with a brush handle produces a:
   a) chip
   b) hollow ring
   c) scratch
   d) clicking sound ____

25. Acrylic nails are kept thinner towards the cuticles, free edge, and sidewalls during acrylic application and:
   a) shaping of the nails
   b) polish application
   c) trimming
   d) acrylic removal ____

26. All acrylic nails need maintenance every:
   a) day
   b) week
   c) two to three weeks
   d) two months ____

27. To smooth out imperfections when applying the final acrylic beads, the brush should:
   a) glide
   b) be wet
   c) be dry
   d) be new ____

28. A backfill procedure removes the grown-out areas and replaces:
   a) a new smile line
   b) an old acrylic nail
   c) a gel nail
   d) a nail tip ____

29. The appointment rotation for any acrylic pink and white French manicure should:
   a) alternate with refill, backfill
   b) alternate with backfill, refill
   c) be performed together every 3 weeks
   d) be alternated every 4 months ____

30. When applying an acrylic nail over a bitten natural nail, before applying the form you must create a:
   a) long free edge
   b) new color powder
   c) bite preventative
   d) part of the nail plate ____

31. The addition of acrylic to the new growth area of the nails is called:
   a) crack repair
   b) fills
   c) lift
   d) polishing ____

32. Without rebalancing, the area near the cuticle, in comparison to the rest of the nail, will be:
   a) lower
   b) whiter
   c) pinker
   d) higher ____

33. The addition of acrylic to reinforce the nail and fill a crack is called:
   a) fill-in
   b) strengthening
   c) crack repair
   d) buffing ____

34. Attempting acrylic removal with nippers can seriously damage the natural nail:
   a) free edge
   b) plate
   c) cuticle
   d) root ____

35. Acrylic products which do not smell as strongly as traditional acrylic products are called:
   a) old
   b) contaminated
   c) polymers
   d) odorless ____

36. When odorless nails are dry, the top surface forms a layer that is
   a) tacky
   b) smooth
   c) rough
   d) oily ____

37. With odorless acrylic, the outer surface once dried can be removed using the manufactured cleaner or:
   a) acetone polish remover
   b) non-acetone polish remover
   c) water and vinegar mixture:
   d) antiseptic ____

38. When filing odorless acrylic products, you should file:
   a) as in traditional acrylics
   b) one direction, toward the free edge
   c) across the nail
   d) toward the cuticle area ____

39. Light cured acrylics are similar to:
   a) gel nails
   b) wraps
   c) odorless acrylics
   d) traditional acrylics ____

40. The dipping method uses cyanoacrylate, which is a fast-setting:
   a) acrylic
   b) catalyst
   c) glue
   d) resin ____

GELS

1. The U.V. gel and nail plate bond together as:
   a) one piece
   b) 2 distinct bonds
   c) 3 distinct bonds
   d) 4 distinct bonds
   ____

2. Each layer of gel requires exposure under:
   a) an electric nail dryer
   b) infrared lights
   c) U.V. light
   d) manicuring light
   ____

3. Colored gels make a good base for:
   a) nail tips
   b) acrylic nails
   c) nail art
   d) the top coat
   ____

4. Gel is applied by brushing on to the:
   a) free edge
   b) entire nail
   c) lunula
   d) cuticle
   ____

5. Gel #2 or building gel is applied:
   a) down the center of the nail
   b) across the free edge of
      the nail
   c) from side to side
      on the nail
   d) from the free edge
      toward the cuticle
   ____

6. For most gel applications:
   a) a primer is required
   b) removing the natural shine
      is not required
   c) a primer is not
      required
   d) sanitation is not
      required
   ____

7. To remove the tacky residue from the nail, the cleaner is
   usually acetone-based or:
   a) acid-based
   b) water-based
   c) alkaline-based
   d) alcohol
   ____

8. The entire nail surface is vigorously buffed:
   a) before the basecoat
   b) before the second coat
   c) before the procedure
      begins
   d) before the topcoat
   ____

9. The type of gel nails that do not require the use of the U.V.
   light is known as:
   a) dipping gels
   b) water gels
   c) no-light gels
   d) curing gels
   ____

10. Gel nails over forms are the best choice for clients who
    want length without:
    a) strength
    b) color
    c) weight
    d) shape
    ____

11. With no-light gels, a second application of gel is often:
    a) time-consuming
    b) dangerous
    c) messy
    d) unnecessary
    ____

12. Gel nails should be maintained every:
   a) week
   b) two to three weeks
   c) two to three months
   d) month
   ____

13. No-light gel nails are removed by soaking nails in:
   a) hydrogen peroxide
   b) alcohol
   c) acetone
   d) water
   ____

14. UV gel nails are removed by:
   a) buffing layer by layer
   b) soaking in water
   c) soaking in acetone
   d) extended exposure to UV light
   ____

15. During gel maintenance, when filing the hardened gel and the natural nail plate you should hold the file:
   a) at a 45° angle
   b) at a 35° angle
   c) flat
   d) at a 90° angle
   ____

chapter 18

THE CREATIVE TOUCH

1. When performing nail art you should:
   a) allow 30 minutes for each appointment
   b) allow ample time
   c) allow 10 minutes per nail
   d) schedule as a regular manicure service ____

2. A display of your nail art will:
   a) generate interest in your services
   b) make co-workers respect you
   c) clutter your work area
   d) make you look unprofessional ____

3. Unless specifically directed before applying some types of nail art, the polish should be:
   a) left damp
   b) applied after designs
   c) completely dry
   d) applied between art applications ____

4. When certain forms of dimensional art are applied to an unstable surface, it will yield:
   a) undesired results
   b) a new art dimension
   c) desired results
   d) a satisfied customer ____

5. To seal in artwork you should:
   a) brush the nail surface
   b) dip the nail in glue
   c) drop a bead of sealer onto the nail surface
   d) not worry about sealing ____

6. Art work such as foiling should be priced by:
   a) the cost of the material
   b) time investment
   c) general availability
   d) a, b, and c ____

7. When the brush floats on the surface of the sealer but never contacts the surface, this is referred to as:
   a) brushing the bead
   b) floating the bead
   c) moving the bead
   d) manipulating the bead ____

8. Pure colors that cannot be obtained from mixing any other colors together are known as:
   a) secondary colors
   b) tertiary colors
   c) complementary colors
   d) primary colors ____

9. The primary colors include all except:
   a) red
   b) yellow
   c) blue
   d) green ____

10. Colors resulting from mixing equal parts of two primary colors together form:
   a) secondary colors
   b) teriary colors
   c) complementary colors
   d) primary colors _____

11. Secondary colors include all except:
   a) blue
   b) violet
   c) range
   d) green _____

12. Colors developed by mixing equal parts of one primary color and one of its nearest secondary colors are:
   a) primary colors
   b) secondary colors
   c) tertiary colors
   d) complementary colors _____

13. Colors located directly across from each other on the color wheel are:
   a) primary colors
   b) secondary colors
   c) tertiary colors
   d) complementary colors _____

14. A neutral muddy brown is made by mixing equal parts of all:
   a) primary colors
   b) secondary colors
   c) tertiary colors
   d) complementary colors _____

15. When complementary colors are applied side-by-side they:
   a) cancel out each other
   b) enhance each other
   c) look subtle
   d) show harmony _____

16. All colors mixed equally with the absence of light produces:
   a) white
   b) black
   c) blue
   d) brown _____

17. White is not considered a color and is defined as:
   a) the absence of light
   b) the presence of light
   c) the absence of all colors
   d) a universal shade _____

18. Analogous color is:
   a) 2 spaces apart on the color wheel
   b) 3 spaces apart on the color wheel
   c) beside each other on the color wheel
   d) opposite each other on the color wheel _____

19. When applying gems you should apply a dab of topcoat or nail art sealer to:
   a) your orangewood stick
   b) your gem
   c) the nail
   d) your tweezers _____

20. When applying foil, you must **first** polish the nail and allow it to:
   a) remain damp
   b) feel tacky to the touch
   c) remain wet
   d) completely dry _____

21. When applying foil, the shiny side should be:
   a) facing down
   b) facing up
   c) facing in either direction
   d) removed before application _____

22. The most popular colors in striping tape include all except:
   a) black
   b) blue
   c) silver
   d) gold _____

23. In order to maintain a good seal and a high gloss finish, your clients should apply a topcoat to their nails every:
    a) week
    b) day
    c) 3–4 days
    d) 2 weeks
    ____

24. Freehand painting may also be referred to as:
    a) dimensional nail art
    b) leafing
    c) polishing the nails
    d) flat nail art
    ____

25. The area of the brush where the bristles meet the ferrule is called the:
    a) heel of the brush
    b) belly of the brush
    c) chisel edge
    d) toe
    ____

26. The most common and versatile brush used in freehand painting is the:
    a) flat brush
    b) fan brush
    c) round brush
    d) bright brush
    ____

27. The flat brush is referred to as a:
    a) shader brush
    b) round brush
    c) bright brush
    d) liner brush
    ____

28. The spotter brush is also known as a/an:
    a) outliner
    b) shadow
    c) detailer
    d) airbrush
    ____

29. The three basic brush strokes include all except:
    a) pressure
    b) friction
    c) position
    d) pull
    ____

30. A popular salon service that is considered more attractive and easier to perform when done by airbrushing is the:
    a) clear polish application
    b) leafing effect
    c) plain manicure
    d) french manicure
    ____

chapter 19

SALON BUSINESS

1. The nail care industry annually does business of
   approximately:
   a) $1 million
   b) $5 million
   c) $2 billion
   d) $6 billion
   ____

2. The average full-service salon may employ this many nail
   technicians:
   a) one
   b) three
   c) five
   d) seven
   ____

3. A disadvantage of full-service salons for the nail
   technician is:
   a) hair care
   b) skin care
   c) not enough clients
   d) no backup for sick
   days or vacation
   ____

4. In a nails-only salon, you have the opportunity to interact
   with other technicians as well as the potential to:
   a) increase your business
   b) be exposed to germs
   c) breathe toxic fumes
   d) learn hair care
   ____

5. Payment for services rendered is known as:
   a) compensation
   b) tips
   c) taxes
   d) expenses
   ____

6. When the salon pays you a percentage of the dollars
   generated for the salon you are receiving:
   a) hourly wage
   b) salary
   c) commission
   d) hourly wage plus
   commission
   ____

7. When an individual rents space in a salon this is known as:
   a) commission
   b) booth rental
   c) hourly wage
   d) hourly wage plus
   commission
   ____

8. In a real sense, booth renters own their own business and are responsible
   for:
   a) paying the building rent
   b)paying the utility bills
   c) paying the phone bills
   d) paying for self-
   employment taxes
   ____

9. As a salon employer, the salon owner is responsible for:
   a) withholding all appropriate
   taxes
   b) only paying social security
   c) only withholding
   the federal taxes
   d) only withholding
   state taxes
   ____

10. A conversation between you and a potential employer where information
    is exchanged is called a/an:
    a) consultation
    b) interview
    c) communication process
    d) a message of
    statement
    ____

11. The first impression that a prospective employer has of you is derived from all of the following except:
a) your clothes
b) your make-up
c) your hair
d) your transportation

12. A written summary of your work, academic experience, and qualifications for a job is known as a/an:
a) resume
b) reference
c) interview
d) consultation review

13. People that your potential employer can contact who can attest to your qualifications are known as:
a) references
b) family members
c) referrals
d) point of contacts

14. A letter to the salon interviewer (owner) that tells them why you would like to work in their salon, briefly describes your qualifications, and asks for an interview is called a/an:
a) resume request letter
b) opening letter
c) cover letter
d) information letter

15. After an interview, good follow-up skills should be demonstrated to the prospective employer in the form of a/an:
a) telephone call
b) E-mail
c) a thank-you note
d) unannounced visit

16. The money you make is called:
a) income
b) expenses
c) taxes
d) tips

17. The money you spend is called:
a) allowance
b) outcome
c) withholding
d) expenses

18. Income includes all the following except:
a) salary
b) commissions
c) withholding
d) tips

19. Your expenses working in a salon could include all the following except:
a) car repair
b) equipment
c) supplies
d) professional books/ magazines

20. As a booth renter, you should record each day's schedule in a:
a) master salon appointment book
b) tax record book
c) computer
d) personal appointment calendar

21. To help keep accurate financial records, most salons use a/an:
a) erasable ink pen
b) accounting service
c) honor system
d) duplicate receipt book

22. Daily sales slips, appointment books, and petty cash records are usually kept on file for:
a) one year
b) five years
c) ten years
d) twenty years

23. The payroll book, cancelled checks, monthly and yearly records , and service and inventory records are used in filing tax returns and are normally kept for at least:
    a) two years
    b) five years
    c) seven years
    d) ten years ____

24. Monthly and yearly records can be a valuable resource for:
    a) sheltering income
    b) determining peak and slow months
    c) determining popular services
    d) raising prices ____

25. Daily inventory records help to quickly detect loss of supplies and retail product due to:
    a) theft
    b) heat
    c) cold
    d) expiration dates ____

26. The income you make minus all your expenses is called:
    a) gross pay
    b) withholding
    c) tax deferred
    d) net income ____

27. Records to help compare the use of supplies with services are called:
    a) inventory
    b) material and supply levels
    c) client service records
    d) retail receipts ____

28. The listing of services rendered and products sold to each client is called the:
    a) material level
    b) inventory record
    c) client service record
    d) gross income ____

29. Signed release statements are kept with:
    a) client service records
    b) daily receipts
    c) tax records
    d) the appointment book ____

30. Keeping an accurate record of appointments reduces:
    a) supply waste
    b) paperwork
    c) retail theft
    d) overbooking appointments ____

31. Proper phone etiquette includes:
    a) answering promptly
    b) making clients hold
    c) answering only after six rings
    d) talking in slang ____

32. When scheduling an appointment, be sure to get the client's:
    a) polish preference
    b) credit card number
    c) name and phone number
    d) driver's license number ____

33. To avoid a scheduling error, when taking telephone appointments you should:
    a) never take phone calls
    b) repeat the information to the client
    c) allow time between appointments
    d) call the client back ____

34. To reduce the number of no-shows, it is a good idea to:
    a) call clients to confirm
    b) overbook
    c) charge for missed appointments
    d) cancel if the client is late ____

35. To conclude your service, always ask clients if they:
    a) will pay cash
    b) wear rubber gloves
    c) bite their nails
    d) would like another appointment _____

36. Call your clients to alert them if you are running late by more than:
    a) 10 minutes
    b) 15 minutes
    c) 20 minutes
    d) 30 minutes _____

37. A written description of services and prices is called the:
    a) service contract
    b) service list
    c) referral brochure
    d) job description _____

38. A pricing practice to be avoided is the offering of reduced prices:
    a) to attract clientele
    b) to promote a service
    c) to only selected clients
    d) in a package deal _____

Chapter 20

SELLING NAIL PRODUCTS AND SERVICES

1. Successful nail technicians are skilled professionals and:
   a) very artistic
   b) good at bookkeeping
   c) good salespeople
   d) salon managers ____

2. One of the basic steps in selling is to:
   a) talk fast
   b) know the product
   c) wave hands around
   d) offer the smallest size ____

3. A specific fact about a product or service is called a:
   a) feature
   b) cost base
   c) service point
   d) profit center ____

4. How a product will fulfill your client's needs is called a:
   a) service point
   b) feature
   c) personal chemistry
   d) benefit ____

5. The best nail choice for a cosmetics salesperson may be:
   a) short and polished
   b) medium and buffed
   c) long acrylic
   d) short gel ____

6. The best nail choice for a pianist may be:
   a) short and natural-looking
   b) medium and polished
   c) long acrylic
   d) medium gel with artwork ____

7. For special occasions, a client may want to match their nails with:
   a) their hairstyle
   b) their clothing
   c) their makeup
   d) their pedicure ____

8. One way to sell products is to tell clients about them:
   a) while you work
   b) after they've paid
   c) when scheduling an appointment
   d) when they ask ____

9. To generate interest in your services, prominently display your:
   a) resume
   b) pedicure foot baths
   c) service list
   d) beauty school diploma ____

10. To encourage retail sales, offer your clients all the following except:
    a) product brochures
    b) product attractively displayed
    c) free samples
    d) coffee and cookies ____

11. You should sell your clients the products they need for:
    a) home acrylic application
    b) home nail maintenance
    c) home gel application
    d) home fabric wrap application ____

12. A great way to promote holidays and events throughout the year can be done by creating and using a:
    a) yearly promotional calendar
    b) monthly promotional calendar
    c) weekly promotional calendar
    d) client's birthday calendar ____

13. Do not diminish the value of your services with discounts; instead try:
    a) value-added
    b) increasing your prices
    c) lowering your prices
    d) giving away used products ____

14. If you don't know the answer to a client's question:
    a) pretend that you do
    b) change the subject
    c) refer them to another technician
    d) volunteer to find out ____

15. A client's objection should be answered:
    a) by talking rapidly
    b) rudely
    c) honestly and pleasantly
    d) with sarcasm ____

16. When a client has valid objections to a product or service, you should:
    a) walk away
    b) suggest another option
    c) get angry
    d) refuse them service ____

17. When a client decides to buy a product or service, you have:
    a) closed the sale
    b) out-smarted them
    c) pleased the boss
    d) successfully maneuvered them ____

18. Suggesting products or services for clients to buy is called:
    a) being pushy
    b) retailing
    c) final service
    d) suggestion selling ____

19. You will be successful at suggestion selling when you can match products and services with your client's:
    a) needs and wants
    b) budget
    c) clothing
    d) hairstyle ____

20. When a client makes another appointment, give them a "reminder card" by writing the date and time on your:
    a) scratch pad
    b) 3" x 5" card
    c) business card
    d) pink reminder papers ____

21. Advance scheduling is a good way to:
    a) plan days off
    b) build steady clientele
    c) plan budgets
    d) order supplies ____

22. A client appointment that occurs the same day at the same time is called a/an:
    a) return visit
    b) standing appointment
    c) pre-booking request
    d) hourly appointment ____

23. Your client retention rate measures how many of your clients:
    a) are new clients
    b) are friends
    c) are existing clients
    d) are yearly clients ____

TYPICAL STATE EXAMINATIONS

100 MULTIPLE CHOICE QUESTIONS

Directions: Carefully read each statement. Insert on the blank line after each statement the letter representing the word or phrase that correctly completes the statement.

1. Ultraviolet radiation is harmful to:
   a) bones
   b) nail polish
   c) eyes
   d) acrylic tips ____

2. Liquid acrylic is a type of:
   a) polymer
   b) monomer
   c) catalyst
   d) curing ____

3. A condition in which white spots appear on the nails is called:
   a) leukonychia
   b) atrophy
   c) nevus
   d) super atrophy ____

4. State regulators expect a salon environment to be:
   a) sterile
   b) infectious
   c) decorative
   d) sanitary ____

5. By understanding body structure, you will be more proficient when doing:
   a) fiber wraps
   b) basic manicures
   c) pedicures
   d) hand and arm massage ____

6. All living things are made up of this basic unit, called the:
   a) cell
   b) protein
   c) nucleus
   d) beta blocker ____

7. Bacteria can be found nearly everywhere; there are this many known types:
   a) 15,000
   b) 5,000
   c) 10,000
   d) 1,500 ____

8. This activity is dangerous around nail chemicals:
   a) gossiping
   b) chewing gum
   c) talking loudly
   d) smoking ____

9. This medical specialty focuses on skin problems:
   a) cardiology
   b) dermatology
   c) esthetics
   d) podiatry ____

10. A client consultation is the conversation you have with the client before:
a) starting the service
b) they make an appointment
c) they pay
d) they buy retail products _____

11. The manicure table should have a bulb of this wattage in the lamp:
a) 60
b) 100
c) 40
d) 150 _____

12. Natural immunity is obtained by keeping the body:
a) warm
b) healthy
c) underweight
d) overweight _____

13. The condition in which the nail loosens from the nail bed is:
a) paronychia
b) oncophagy
c) onychia
d) onycholysis _____

14. Sculptured nails are also known as:
a) acrylic nails
b) manicured nails
c) nail wraps
d) extra long nails _____

15. The recommended maintenance schedule for all acrylic nails is every:
a) month
b) two to three weeks
c) day
d) six months _____

16. Your sense of right and wrong when you interact with clients, employer, and coworkers is called:
a) honesty
b) professional ethics
c) moral values
d) moodiness _____

17. Massage, nerve impulses, and light rays are some of the ways to stimulate:
a) phalanges
b) muscles
c) sanitation
d) eyes _____

18. The muscles which can cause goose bumps are called the:
a) arrector pili
b) papillae
c) goosli muscles
d) lesion _____

19. An emery board is an example of an item that is:
a) wet sanitized
b) heat sanitized
c) disposable
d) purchased individually _____

20. If the nail tip covers the nail plate from sidewall to sidewall, it is:
a) too wide
b) properly sized
c) too long
d) too narrow _____

21. The French Manicure look can be created through the:
a) one-color acrylic method
b) proper diet
c) proper buffing techniques
d) two-color acrylic method _____

22. In acrylic applications, the free edge is formed with the:
a) first acrylic ball
b) third acrylic ball
c) nail file
d) second acrylic ball _____

23. Glue should be stored at room temperature between:
    a) 60–85 degrees Celsius
    b) 70–90 degrees Celsius
    c) 60–85 degrees Fahrenheit
    d) 70–90 degrees Fahrenheit ____

24. Soft or fragile nails should be filed using a/an:
    a) emery board
    b) metal nail file
    c) chamois buffer
    d) nail brush ____

25. Hypoallergenic products are used for the client's:
    a) pharmacist
    b) skin cancer
    c) safety
    d) acne ____

26. The movements of the body are controlled by the:
    a) efferent nerves
    b) peripheral system
    c) blood
    d) central nervous system ____

27. When conditions are unfavorable for reproduction, bacteria will go dormant after forming a tough covering called a:
    a) shell
    b) mitosis
    c) spore
    d) flagella ____

28. Non-acetone remover is used to remove polish from:
    a) hangnails
    b) artificial tips
    c) toenails
    d) accidental spills on clothing ____

29. A repair patch is a piece of fabric cut to:
    a) the nail's shape
    b) $1/4$ inch by $1/4$ inch
    c) completely cover a crack or break
    d) $1/2$ inch by $1/2$ inch ____

30. Insomnia, watery eyes, and sluggishness are symptoms of chemical:
    a) overexposure
    b) inhalation
    c) burn
    d) poisoning ____

31. In order to have a good working relationship with coworkers, you should:
    a) respect their opinions
    b) use deodorant
    c) buy their lunch
    d) point out mistakes ____

32. Liquid nail wrap is used to:
    a) speed the silk wrap procedure
    b) preserve nail art
    c) strengthen natural nail
    d) cover fungi ____

33. The opaqueness of linen wraps requires that they be covered with:
    a) glitter
    b) mending tissue
    c) clear polish
    d) colored polish ____

34. Always refuse service and refer a client to a physician if they have a skin or nail:
    a) hangnail
    b) inflammation
    c) bruise
    d) callus ____

35. Tanning is caused by exposing skin to the sun's:
    a) ultraviolet rays
    b) keratoma
    c) vitamin D
    d) carotene ____

36. Learning about other services offered at the salon, such as hair and skin care, and then telling your clients about them, is called salon:
    a) performance
    b) showoff
    c) networking
    d) promotion ____

37. In acrylic nails, the transfer of heat until the last polymer receives heat is known as:
    a) cold reaction
    b) dehydration
    c) polymerization
    d) catalyst ____

38. The best way to protect yourself and your clients against infection is to always:
    a) ask if they have an infection
    b) wear masks
    c) sanitize implements properly
    d) sit at arm's length ____

39. Mending liquid is a heavy adhesive used to apply:
    a) silk wraps
    b) paper wraps
    c) linen wraps
    d) nail gems ____

40. To remove acrylic nails, they should be soaked in:
    a) non-acetone polish remover
    b) brush cleaner
    c) water
    d) acetone polish remover ____

41. The technical name for callus is:
    a) freckle
    b) stratum lucidum
    c) tyloma
    d) mole ____

42. Bacilli and spirilla propel themselves with hairlike projections known as:
    a) flagella
    b) propellants
    c) mitosis
    d) cocci ____

43. To protect hands and nails when doing housework, clients should wear:
    a) silicone lotion
    b) rubber gloves
    c) clear polish
    d) a dust mask ____

44. Linen wraps:
    a) are thicker than silk
    b) do not last long
    c) are considered a thin wrap
    d) are loosely woven ____

45. The nerve which supplies impulses to the top of the foot is the:
    a) dorsal
    b) digital
    c) saphenous
    d) ulnar ____

46. Unsanitary implements can cause these nail disorders:
    a) onychomycosis
    b) mold
    c) onychia and paronychia
    d) nevus ____

47. Cuticle pushers are also known as:
    a) nippers
    b) oils
    c) emery boards
    d) steel pushers ____

48. The most common nail shape for male clients is:
    a) square
    b) oval
    c) round
    d) pointed ____

49. To prevent contamination of the disinfectant, disinfection containers should be kept:
a) warm c) cold
b) covered d) in cupboards ____

50. Client service records are usually kept on:
a) pink paper c) triplicate forms
b) blue paper d) index cards ____

51. Foot files are used to remove:
a) warts c) callus growths
b) hangnails d) fungus ____

52. Eyes can be damaged by improperly shielded:
a) ultraviolet lamps c) polish
b) fingerbowls d) autoclaves ____

53. The lowest level of decontamination is:
a) sterilization c) disinfections
b) sanitation d) washing ____

54. An example of an employee benefit would be any of the following except:
a) medical insurance c) paid parking space
b) life insurance d) earning minimum wage ____

55. Your personal problems should always be:
a) shared with coworkers c) left at home
b) shared with clients d) told to the boss ____

56. A client with athlete's foot may not receive:
a) a pedicure c) colored polish
b) a foot massage d) pedicure slippers ____

57. To draw with an airbrush, you need to use a/an:
a) orangewood stick c) sponge
b) design tool d) nail pen ____

58. On an annual basis, the nail care industry annually does this much business:
a) $3 billion c) $6 billion
b) $5 million d) $10 million ____

59. A common condition in which the cuticle around the nail splits is known as:
a) a hangnail c) nail crack
b) skin overgrowth d) a callus ____

60. Prevent chemical accidents by never using a product if the container is not:
a) sealed c) full
b) sanitized d) labeled ____

61. It is dangerous to judge if a chemical is safe by its:
a) label c) ingredients
b) odor d) MSDS ____

62. Clear, white, and pink are colors of:
    a) acrylic powder
    b) sable brushes
    c) toe separators
    d) paper towels _____

63. The tacky feel of the surface of odorless acrylic nails indicates the nails are:
    a) old
    b) separating from the nail plate
    c) dry
    d) needing a fill _____

64. This layer of epidermis has cells that look like granules:
    a) stratum corneum
    b) stratum mucosum
    c) stratum lucidum
    d) stratum granulosum _____

65. Nails which are thin, white, and curved over the free edge are called:
    a) furrowed
    b) normal
    c) eggshell
    d) dry _____

66. Color and gloss is added to the nail through the application of:
    a) colored polish
    b) a silk wrap
    c) buffing compound
    d) mending liquid _____

67. During gel nail procedures, the entire nail surface is vigorously brushed to smooth the finish before:
    a) beginning the service
    b) the nads are sanitized
    c) you apply the topcoat
    d) you apply the basecoat _____

68. Formalin contains formaldehyde which causes the following except:
    a) muscle pain
    b) lung irritation
    c) rash
    d) skin irritation _____

69. To make them feel welcome, new clients should be:
    a) greeted by name
    b) given a salon tour
    c) escorted to a station
    d) all the above _____

70. Most pedicure services are performed by starting with:
    a) right foot, little toe
    b) right foot, middle toe
    c) left foot, little toe
    d) left foot, big toe _____

71. The client who wants length without weight should receive:
    a) paper wraps
    b) gel nails
    c) linen wraps
    d) silk wraps _____

72. To give sparkle to a nail art design, use:
    a) gems
    b) metallic polish
    c) sequins
    d) a fine buffer block _____

73. If the nail or skin to be worked on is inflamed, broken, swollen, or infected, the client must:
    a) be sanitized with alcohol
    b) be referred to a physician
    c) need a manicure
    d) scrub with soap _____

74. Expenses are defined as the money you:
    a) earn
    b) save
    c) spend
    d) donate _____

75. A technician who is a good salesperson and a skilled professional will also be:
    a) artistic
    b) a good receptionist
    c) a good manager
    d) very successful _____

76. A client may want to match nails with clothing for a/an:
    a) special occasion
    b) few days
    c) few weeks
    d) entire year _____

77. The "true skin" is the deep layer of skin which is called the:
    a) cuticle
    b) cutis
    c) epidermis
    d) clavicle _____

78. The heat from warm paraffin wax:
    a) closes the skin pores
    b) helps the polish to last longer
    c) moisturizes the skin
    d) helps cure gel when applied _____

79. If a chemical agent gets on your clothing, immediately:
    a) dab with water
    b) blot with a towel
    c) use spot remover
    d) remove the garment _____

80. Natural nails can be lengthened by adding:
    a) artificial tips
    b) silk wraps
    c) paper wraps
    d) nail art _____

81. A primer is applied to the natural nail in order for the acrylic product to:
    a) dry properly
    b) polish easily
    c) adhere
    d) prevent fungus _____

82. A long acrylic nail may be the best choice for a woman who is a:
    a) guitar player
    b) pianist
    c) gardener
    d) cosmetic salesperson _____

83. Dry cuticles can cause:
    a) nail biting
    b) buffing problems
    c) hangnails
    d) wraps to lift _____

84. Most clients are relaxed by:
    a) effleurage
    b) clear polish applications
    c) thumb compression
    d) metatarsal scissors _____

85. Seven years is the amount of time you should keep business records which were used to:
    a) pay off loans
    b) complete tax returns
    c) pay employees
    d) order supplies _____

86. An acquired superficial, round, and thickened patch of epidermis due to pressure or friction on the hands or feet is called:
    a) cocci
    b) eczema
    c) tyloma
    d) flagella _____

87. Fabric wraps are not a good service choice for a client whose hands are frequently:
    a) in gloves
    b) held
    c) photographed
    d) in water _____

88. Peak and slow months can be determined by reviewing your:
    a) monthly records
    b) tax withholding
    c) customer list
    d) supply inventory _____

89. A liquid that kills or retards bacterial growth is a/an:
    a) soap
    b) solution
    c) antiseptic
    d) agent _____

90. When applying acrylic over nail tips, you do not need to use a/an:
    a) acrylic powder
    b) sable brush
    c) acrylic liquid
    d) nail form ____

91. Chemical storage should be in cool areas and away from:
    a) any appliance/furnace with a pilot light
    b) hair colors
    c) perm solutions
    d) garbage cans ____

92. To add shine to the nail, use a chamois buffer with pumice powder or:
    a) water
    b) cuticle oil
    c) dry polish
    d) cuticle remover ____

93. An accounting service is often used to help salons keep:
    a) making a profit
    b) accurate financial records
    c) making loan payments
    d) tax losses large ____

94. A catalyst is an ingredient which causes a process to:
    a) explode
    b) slow down
    c) speed up
    d) remain static ____

95. Sebum is secreted by:
    a) seals
    b) oil glands
    c) arteries
    d) infected skin ____

96. Plastic gloves and safety glasses should always be worn when working with:
    a) primers
    b) gel nails
    c) air brushes
    d) acrylic powders ____

97. Another name for a wart is:
    a) tubercle
    b) wheal
    c) papilloma
    d) vesicle ____

98. The skin's outer layer is called the:
    a) dermis
    b) epidermis
    c) subcutaneous tissue
    d) stratum corneum ____

99. The proper way to mix polish is to:
    a) mix it with top coat
    b) shake vigorously
    c) tap the bottle on a table
    d) roll the bottle between your palms ____

100. A weekly reconditioning hot oil manicure will benefit clients with:
    a) dry cuticles
    b) gel nails
    c) paper wraps
    d) arthritis ____

Directions: Carefully read each statement. Insert on the blank line after each statement the letter representing the word or phrase that correctly completes the statement.

1. Two-color acrylic application requires use of all the following except:
   a) white tip powder   c) pink powder
   b) yellow powder   d) acrylic liquid   ____

2. The common name for onychocryptosis is:
   a) hangnail   c) ingrown nail
   b) nail biting   d) bruise   ____

3. Spraying nail antiseptic on nails removes:
   a) cotton bits   c) nail filings
   b) polish   d) natural oil   ____

4. Artificial enhancements are examples of coating created by:
   a) a physical reaction   c) a combination reaction
   b) a chemical reaction   d) a chemical restriction ____

5. The largest system in the body is the:
   a) skeletal   c) circulatory
   b) integumentary   d) digestive   ____

6. The chemicals from nail products enter your body in all these ways except:
   a) inhalation   c) injection
   b) ingestion   d) skin contact   ____

7. If pus is present, the skin or nail is:
   a) infected   c) bruised
   b) to be soaked in alcohol d) inflamed   ____

8. Even though nails seem to be a dry hard plate, their water content is:
   a) 15–35%   c) 10–30%
   b) 25–40%   d) 50–60%   ____

9. An important part of the consultation is to determine whether or not the home maintenance for a service fits the client's:
   a) looks   c) budget
   b) lifestyle   d) ability   ____

10. Equipment is the term for items used in nail technology that are:
    a) expensive   c) disposable
    b) made of plastic   d) permanent   ____

11. When pedicuring, the proper time to insert toe separators is before:
    a) clipping the nails   c) filing the nails
    b) polishing the nails   d) soaking the feet   ____

12. The foot massage begins with:
    a) joint relaxer movements
    b) thumb compression
    c) metatarsal scissors
    d) brisk rubbing _____

13. Bacteria multiply at amazing speeds—in only half a day, a single bacteria cell can produce this many more:
    a) 6,000
    b) 16 million
    c) 100,000
    d) 25,000 _____

14. Albinism is the congenital absence of this substance from the body:
    a) albumin
    b) fungus
    c) melanin
    d) Vitamin C _____

15. Performing a service on an infected nail could cause your client a great deal of:
    a) healing
    b) pain
    c) regrowth
    d) filing _____

16. Phenolics are good for implement disinfection but are:
    a) difficult to work with
    b) unbalanced
    c) hard to find
    d) costly _____

17. Your best source of advertising to attract new clients is:
    a) radio
    b) current satisfied clients
    c) newspapers
    d) coupon mailers _____

18. A lamp bulb with high wattage will affect product performance when giving this service:
    a) sculptured nails
    b) gel nails
    c) polish change
    d) fiber wrap _____

19. The body is protected from harmful infection and bacteria through the white cells found in:
    a) urine
    b) blood
    c) sebum
    d) skin _____

20. A properly ventilated salon is one that vents fumes and vapors to the:
    a) reception area
    b) bathroom
    c) outside
    d) haircolor area _____

21. Black bands seen under or within the nail plate are known as:
    a) plicatured
    b) verruca
    c) onychophagy
    d) melanonychia _____

22. To avoid ingrown toenails, file the nails straight across with:
    a) steel implements
    b) slightly rounded corners
    c) metal files
    d) chamois buffers _____

23. Healthy nails result from:
    a) a general state of health
    b) regular trimming
    c) eating bananas
    d) drinking carrot juice _____

24. Fingernails grow faster than:
    a) hair
    b) bones
    c) toenails
    d) muscles _____

25. Paper wraps will dissolve in:
    a) water
    b) dishwashing liquid
    c) polish applications
    d) polish remover _____

26. To reseal wrap during a glue fill, apply adhesive to:
    a) any broken edges
    b) the polish brush before application
    c) the entire nail
    d) only the thumb nails   ____

27. Finished acrylic nails are:
    a) polymers
    b) monomers
    c) polymerizations
    d) catalysts   ____

28. Foil leaf is available in gold, silver, and:
    a) bronze
    b) copper
    c) turquoise
    d) onyx   ____

29. Nonpathogenic bacteria belong to the group of bacteria known as:
    a) spirilla
    b) viruses
    c) cocci
    d) saprophytes   ____

30. Problems or questions about your job should be discussed with:
    a) your co-workers
    b) your best friend
    c) your employer
    d) your mother   ____

31. To ensure full potency, chemical agents for sanitation should be purchased:
    a) in bulk
    b) in small quantities
    c) by mail
    d) on sunny days   ____

32. If no overlay is applied, an artificial tip is very:
    a) weak
    b) colorful
    c) apparent
    d) natural-looking   ____

33. A small elevation above the skin surface that has a solid center and can be felt is known as a/an:
    a) macule
    b) bulla
    c) scale
    d) papule   ____

34. Overlay is another name for:
    a) stencils
    b) nail wraps
    c) gem applications
    d) gel applications   ____

35. The joints in the ankle and wrist are known as:
    a) ball joints
    b) cartilage
    c) gliding joints
    d) carpus   ____

36. Extra long natural nails are not suited for this service:
    a) paper wraps
    b) reconditioning hot oil manicure
    c) French Manicure
    d) nail art   ____

37. Percussion movements are also called:
    a) drum symphonies
    b) tapotement movements
    c) tingle toes
    d) tapping touches   ____

38. In acrylic technique, when the sable brush is dipped into liquid, then powder, this forms:
    a) glue
    b) a chalky white color
    c) baking soda
    d) an acrylic ball   ____

39. Store acrylic products:
    a) on well-lit shelves
    b) near the manicure lamp
    c) in covered containers
    d) near a heating unit   ____

40. An MSDS can be obtained from your salon's:
    a) distributor
    c) cleaning person
    b) main office
    d) fire department ____

41. The deep layer of skin is called the:
    a) epidermis
    c) subcutaneous layer
    b) dermis
    d) nutrient level ____

42. An orangewood stick is classified as a/an:
    a) nail file
    c) implement
    b) equipment
    d) reusable item ____

43. The free edge of sculptured nails should be shaped with a/an:
    a) tweezer
    c) chamois buffer
    b) cuticle nipper
    d) metal nail file ____

44. Striping tape is used to create lines when doing:
    a) football field markings
    c) toenail clipping
    b) nail art
    d) a French Manicure ____

45. Onychauxis is the technical term for a nail's:
    a) overgrowth
    c) bruise
    b) infection
    d) removal ____

46. Chloasma is commonly known as:
    a) freckles
    c) liver spots
    b) birthmark
    d) tanning ____

47. An accidental splash of solvent or primer can seriously injure the:
    a) nail
    c) implements
    b) polish
    d) eyes ____

48. Manicure friction massage involves a wringing movement on the:
    a) toe
    c) fingers
    b) arm
    d) wrist ____

49. When removing artificial tips, first soak them in remover to:
    a) dissolve the free edge
    c) soften them
    b) remove the polish
    d) dissolve the sidewalls ____

50. The chalky white color of primer during acrylic application indicates the primer is:
    a) dry
    c) old
    b) odorless
    d) not properly mixed ____

51. The essential oil that is stimulating to circulation, relieves pain, and is a decongestant is:
    a) cypress
    c) bergamot
    b) rosemary
    d) tea tree ____

52. The number of nerve endings found in the feet is more than:
    a) 500
    c) 5,000
    c) 10,000
    d) 50,000 ____

53. Odorless acrylics are self-leveling, which means they require less:
    a) product
    c) shaping
    b) brushing
    d) buffing ____

54. Consumable supplies are the supplies used to:
    a) provide services
    c) stock retail kits
    b) give as samples
    d) eat lunch ____

55. Short and natural-looking is the best nail choice for a person who is a:
a) computer operator   c) pianist
b) telephone receptionist   d) stockbroker   ____

56. A good way to develop a steady clientele is to ask clients, before they leave the salon, to:
a) buy retail   c) wash their hands
b) make another appointment   d) select polish   ____

57. The large, thick triangular muscle that covers the shoulder and lifts and turns the arm is called the:
a) armature   c) chloasma
b) turner   d) deltoid   ____

58. Because of the chemical hazards, a child present at your work station should be properly:
a) supervised   c) rested
b) fed   d) clothed   ____

59. The muscle which turns the hand outward so the palm faces upward is called the:
a) terminator   c) pronator
b) supinator   d) fibula   ____

60. Onyx is the technical term for:
a) hair   c) nails
b) skin   d) eyes   ____

61. Net income is the money you make less all your:
a) expenses   c) clothes
b) groceries   d) income   ____

62. Orange, green, and violet colors are known as:
a) complimentary colors   c) primary colors
b) tertiary colors   d) secondary colors   ____

63. Clear cells are found in the skin layer called:
a) stratum corneum   c) melanin
b) stratum lucidum   d) stratum mucosum   ____

64. A written description of services and prices is called the:
a) job description   c) service list
b) promotions ad   d) contract   ____

65. A light-colored, slightly raised mark on the skin formed after an injury or lesion of the skin has healed is called a/an:
a) scar   c) abrasion
b) scratch   d) callus   ____

66. The practice of offering only selected clients reduced prices should be:
a) done discreetly   c) encouraged
b) a weekly ritual   d) avoided   ____

67. Acrylic nails must be removed by soaking fingertips in:
a) acetone   c) cuticle remover
b) baby oil   d) alcohol   ____

68. Pure pigmented colors that cannot be obtained from mixing any other colors together are:
a) complementary
b) tertiary
c) primary
d) secondary
____

69. No backup when you are gone is a disadvantage of working in:
a) a nails-only salon
b) a full-service salon
c) your own salon
d) selected areas
____

70. Problems generally associated with nail thickness as well as some surface irregularities of the plate are:
a) nail plate disorders
b) circulation problems
c) matrix bad problems
d) digestion problems
____

71. The clicking sound made by gently tapping the brush handle on an applied acrylic nail indicates the nails:
a) are dry
b) are cracking
c) are new
d) need replacing
____

72. Honesty is the best policy when dealing with a client's:
a) polish
b) objections
c) nail file
d) pedicure
____

73. Income is the:
a) money you make
b) incoming client
c) money you spend
d) taxes due
____

74. To speed the filing of long nails, first shorten them with a:
a) nail buffer
b) metal nail file
c) fingernail clipper
d) emery board
____

75. The fingerbowl used during a manicure contains water and:
a) alcohol
b) antibacterial soap
c) fungicide
d) fumigants
____

76. Metatarsal scissors is a massage movement which promotes:
a) blood flow to the neck
b) blood flow to the legs
c) cutting ability
d) flexibility
____

77. An easy way for a nail technician to earn additional income is through:
a) retail sales
b) double-booking clients
c) cleaning houses
d) changing professions
____

78. The nail unit that is composed of matrix cells and produces the nail plate is the:
a) hyponychium
b) eponychium
c) matrix bed
d) lunula
____

79. An airbrush can be used with colored polish in nail art to create:
a) shades and textures
b) quick designs
c) translucent applications
d) a gel nails base
____

80. A temporary artificial nail service is a:
a) mending job
b) demonstration service
c) tip with no overlay
d) tip applied with water glue
____

81. Rotation of the elbow is a type of:
    a) chiropractic manipulation   c) effleurage
    b) friction massage movement   d) relaxer movement   _____

82. By spraying the client's nails with water, you can reduce the heat
    generated during:
    a) buffing   c) polishing
    b) acrylic removal   d) filing   _____

83. The half-moon shape at the base of the nail is called the:
    a) mantle   c) lunula
    b) matrix   d) groove   _____

84. An advantage of quats as a sanitation agent is their:
    a) stability   c) odor
    b) weak solution   d) bacteria   _____

85. This substance can be found in the stratum germinativum layer
    of the epidermis:
    a) elasticity   c) herpes simplex
    b) mold   d) melanin   _____

86. The service of trimming, shaping, and polishing toenails, as well
    as performing foot massage, is called:
    a) podiatry   c) pedicuring
    b) manicuring   d) filing   _____

87. Circular movements in the palm is a massage technique known as:
    a) effleurage   c) friction massage
    b) tapping   d) joint relaxer
                                           movements   _____

88. Only half of the nail plate should be covered by a/an:
    a) glitter polish   c) French Manicure polish
       application   d) buffer block
    b) artificial nail tip   _____

89. Crack repair of an acrylic nail is performed using:
    a) silk wrap   c) acrylic
    b) mending tissue   d) clear polish   _____

90. The epidermis contains no:
    a) cells   c) nerves
    b) blood vessels   d) keratin   _____

91. Questions about a client's job are part of the:
    a) health information   c) friendship process
    b) service record   d) client profile   _____

92. The client's circulation is stimulated by:
    a) massage   c) buffing
    b) tip application   d) filing   _____

93. Tuberculocidal disinfectants are required to clean:
    a) toilet seats   c) the bathroom floor
    b) visible blood spills   d) cuticle nippers   _____

94. A combination build-up of bed epithelium and hyponychial tissue
    is known as the:
    a) onychodermal band   c) eponychium band
    b) nail band   d) proximal band   _____

95. The excess skin beneath a toenail's free edge may be softened by using:
    a) alcohol
    b) silicone lotion
    c) cuticle solvent
    d) polish remover
    ____

96. To avoid smearing polish, especially in a pedicure application, the top coat should be followed by:
    a) nail strengthener
    b) a second top coat
    c) hot blowing air
    d) instant nail dry
    ____

97. Ridges that are created when using a bit at the wrong angle at the cuticle area are known as:
    a) lunulas
    b) rings of fire
    c) onychodermal bands
    d) proximal rings
    ____

98. Always begin a manicure by working with the client's hand that is:
    a) not the favored one
    b) favored one
    c) in worse shape
    d) closest
    ____

99. Skin that is red and sore is called:
    a) healthy
    b) infected
    c) inflamed
    d) circulated
    ____

100. RPM stands for:
    a) revolutions per minute
    b) revolutions per month
    c) revolutions per machine
    d) regular pressure machine
    ____

ANSWERS TO EXAM REVIEW FOR NAIL TECHNOLOGY

YOUR PROFESSIONAL IMAGE

1-c	6-a	11-b	16-b	21-d	26-b
2-b	7-d	12-a	17-b	22-a	27-b
3-b	8-a	13-c	18-c	23-c	28-a
4-a	9-d	14-c	19-a	24-b	29-d
5-c	10-b	15-d	20-a	25-c	30-c

BACTERIA AND OTHER INFECTIOUS AGENTS

1-d	6-d	11-d	16-d	21-a	26-a	31-c	36-b
2-b	7-a	12-a	17-a	22-c	27-c	32-b	37-c
3-c	8-d	13-c	18-c	23-d	28-d	33-d	38-c
4-b	9-b	14-b	19-b	24-b	29-a	34-b	
5-c	10-c	15-a	20-d	25-d	30-a	35-d	

SANITATION AND DISINFECTION

1-a	6-d	11-c	16-d	21-d	26-c
2-d	7-c	12-c	17-c	22-c	27-a
3-b	8-a	13-b	18-b	23-b	28-c
4-c	9-c	14-b	19-c	24-b	29-b
5-b	10-a	15-a	20-d	25-d	30-a

SAFETY IN THE SALON

1-c	6-d	11-b	16-c	21-c	26-d	31-b
2-b	7-a	12-b	17-d	22-b	27-a	32-b
3-d	8-d	13-b	18-a	23-d	28-b	33-a
4-b	9-c	14-c	19-a	24-b	29-d	34-a
5-a	10-c	15-c	20-d	25-a	30-c	

NAIL PRODUCT CHEMISTRY SIMPLIFIED

1-a	6-d	11-d	16-a	21-b	26-a	31-c
2-c	7-c	12-d	17-c	22-a	27-c	
3-b	8-a	13-d	18-b	23-c	28-d	
4-d	9-b	14-c	19-b	24-c	29-d	
5-b	10-a	15-b	20-d	25-b	30-a	

ANATOMY AND PHYSIOLOGY

1-b	8-a	15-c	22-c	29-d	36-a	43-b
2-c	9-c	16-b	23-b	30-b	37-c	44-a
3-a	10-b	17-d	24-b	31-d	38-c	45-d
4-d	11-d	18-a	25-c	32-a	39-a	
5-b	12-b	19-a	26-a	33-b	40-c	
6-d	13-c	20-d	27-d	34-b	41-b	
7-c	14-a	21-a	28-b	35-a	42-c	

THE NAIL AND ITS DISORDERS

1-b	9-b	17-c	25-a	33-b	41-a	49-c
2-a	10-d	18-d	26-b	34-a	42-d	50-b
3-d	11-c	19-c	27-a	35-c	43-b	
4-d	12-a	20-b	28-c	36-b	44-a	
5-d	13-d	21-d	29-d	37-a	45-c	
6-c	14-a	22-a	30-a	38-a	46-c	
7-b	15-a	23-a	31-a	39-a	47-b	
8-b	16-c	24-b	32-d	40-a	48-d	

THE SKIN AND ITS DISORDERS

1-b	7-b	13-c	19-c	25-b	31-d	37-c
2-c	8-c	14-d	20-b	26-d	32-d	38-d
3-b	9-b	15-b	21-a	27-c	33-a	39-a
4-d	10-a	16-c	22-a	28-b	34-b	40-b
5-c	11-b	17-b	23-b	29-a	35-a	41-c
6-d	12-d	18-a	24-a	30-b	36-b	42-c

CLIENT CONSULTATION

1-b	4-d	7-c	10-a	13-d	16-d
2-d	5-b	8-c	11-a	14-b	17-c
3-c	6-d	9-d	12-c	15-a	18-d

MANICURING

1-b	7-b	13-b	19-c	25-d	31-d	37-b
2-c	8-a	14-c	20-b	26-b	32-a	38-c
3-a	9-c	15-d	21-a	27-d	33-c	39-a
4-c	10-b	16-b	22-b	28-c	34-d	40-d
5-a	11-a	17-d	23-c	29-c	35-d	
6-d	12-d	18-a	24-b	30-a	36-a	

PEDICURING

1-d	7-c	13-a	19-c	25-b	31-b	37-d
2-a	8-d	14-a	20-b	26-d	32-c	
3-b	9-a	15-a	21-a	27-a	33-c	
4-b	10-b	16-b	22-d	28-c	34-a	
5-a	11-d	17-d	23-a	29-b	35-b	
6-b	12-c	18-b	24-c	30-d	36-c	

ELECTRIC FILING

1-d	4-b	7-d	10-b	13-c	16-c	19-d
2-a	5-a	8-c	11-a	14-d	17-a	20-a
3-b	6-b	9-a	12-a	15-c	18-b	21-c

AROMATHERAPY

1-a	4-c	7-a	10-d	13-b
2-d	5-b	8-b	11-a	14-c
3-d	6-b	9-c	12-a	15-d

NAIL TIPS

1-b	6-c	11-b	16-b	21-d	26-c	31-a
2-c	7-b	12-c	17-b	22-a	27-d	
3-b	8-a	13-d	18-b	23-b	28-c	
4-a	9-b	14-a	19-a	24-a	29-b	
5-d	10-d	15-c	20-c	25-c	30-d	

NAIL WRAPS

1-b	6-c	11-a	16-c	21-b	26-c
2-c	7-a	12-d	17-b	22-d	27-a
3-b	8-c	13-c	18-a	23-c	28-b
4-d	9-b	14-b	19-d	24-b	29-c
5-b	10-d	15-a	20-a	25-a	30-d

ACRYLIC NAILS

1-b	7-c	13-c	19-a	25-a	31-b	37-a
2-b	8-a	14-a	20-d	26-c	32-a	38-b
3-b	9-b	15-c	21-b	27-a	33-c	39-c
4-a	10-b	16-d	22-a	28-a	34-b	40-c
5-d	11-c	17-d	23-c	29-b	35-d	
6-d	12-b	18-b	24-d	30-d	36-a	

GELS

1-a	4-b	7-d	10-c	13-d
2-c	5-a	8-d	11-d	14-a
3-c	6-c	9-c	12-b	15-c

THE CREATIVE TOUCH

1-b	6-d	11-a	16-b	21-b	26-c
2-a	7-b	12-c	17-c	22-b	27-a
3-c	8-d	13-d	18-c	23-c	28-c
4-a	9-d	14-d	19-c	24-d	29-b
5-c	10-a	15-b	20-d	25-a	30-d

SALON BUSINESS

1-d	7-b	13-a	19-a	25-a	31-a	37-b
2-a	8-d	14-c	20-d	26-d	32-c	38-c
3-d	9-a	15-c	21-b	27-b	33-b	
4-a	10-b	16-a	22-a	28-c	34-a	
5-a	11-d	17-d	23-c	29-a	35-d	
6-c	12-a	18-c	24-b	30-d	36-b	

SELLING NAIL PRODUCTS AND SERVICES

1-c	5-c	9-c	13-a	17-a	21-b
2-b	6-a	10-d	14-d	18-d	22-b
3-a	7-b	11-b	15-c	19-a	23-c
4-d	8-a	12-a	16-b	20-c	

TEST 1

1-c	16-b	31-a	46-c	61-b	76-a	91-a
2-b	17-b	32-c	47-d	62-a	77-b	92-c
3-a	18-a	33-d	48-c	63-c	78-c	93-b
4-d	19-c	34-b	49-b	64-d	79-d	94-c
5-d	20-b	35-a	50-d	65-c	80-a	95-b
6-a	21-d	36-d	51-c	66-a	81-c	96-a
7-a	22-a	37-c	52-a	67-c	82-d	97-c
8-d	23-c	38-c	53-b	68-a	83-c	98-b
9-b	24-a	39-b	54-d	69-d	84-a	99-d
10-a	25-c	40-d	55-c	70-c	85-b	100-a
11-c	26-d	41-c	56-a	71-b	86-c	
12-b	27-c	42-a	57-b	72-a	87-d	
13-d	28-b	43-b	58-c	73-b	88-a	
14-a	29-c	44-c	59-a	74-c	89-c	
15-b	30-a	45-a	60-d	75-d	90-d	

TEST 2

1-b	16-d	31-b	46-c	61-a	76-d	91-d
2-c	17-b	32-a	47-d	62-d	77-a	92-a
3-d	18-a	33-d	48-b	63-b	78-c	93-b
4-b	19-b	34-b	49-c	65-c	79-a	94-a
5-b	20-c	35-c	50-a	65-a	80-c	95-c
6-c	21-d	36-a	51-b	66-d	81-b	96-d
7-a	22-b	37-b	52-d	67-a	82-a	97-b
8-c	23-a	38-d	53-c	68-c	83-c	98-a
9-b	24-c	39-c	54-a	69-b	84-a	99-c
10-d	25-d	40-a	55-c	70-c	85-d	100-a
11-c	26-c	41-b	56-b	71-a	86-c	
12-a	27-a	42-c	57-d	72-b	87-a	
13-b	28-b	43-d	58-a	73-a	88-b	
14-c	29-d	44-b	59-b	74-c	89-c	
15-b	30-c	45-a	60-c	75-b	90-b	

NOTES

NOTES

NOTES

NOTES

NOTES

NOTES

NOTES

NOTES

NOTES

NOTES

NOTES